AUGUST 2000

Dear Ellen,
a truerfriend there never
was. we will grow old
together and still have
lots to talk about on
our runs. *Love ya*
Gail

IT'S NEVER
TOO LATE !

PERSONAL STORIES OF
STAYING YOUNG THROUGH SPORTS

Gail Waesche Kislevitz

BREAKAWAY BOOKS
HALCOTTSVILLE, NY
2000

It's Never Too Late! Personal Stories of Staying Young Through Sports

Copyright © 2000 by Gail Waesche Kislevitz

ISBN: 1-891369-21-0

Library of Congress Control Number: 00-133190

Published by Breakaway Books
P. O. Box 24
Halcottsville, NY 12438
(800) 548-4348
www.breakawaybooks.com

Breakaway Books are distributed to the trade by Consortium.

FIRST EDITION

To the memory of my parents,
Beatrice Maleady Waesche
and
Donald MacPherson Waesche,
two great examples of how to live life to its fullest.

CONTENTS

ACKNOWLEDGMENTS

A year has gone by since I started this book; a year that has been filled with new ideas and a new outlook on aging. It goes without saying that I could not have written this book without the cooperation and support of the 28 people I interviewed here. They have witnessed the best and worst of the last century and opened their lives to me, sharing stories of love, war, death, and the determination to go on in the face of adversity. These people became my inspiration as well as my friends. Each one is an example of successful aging. They are creative, challenged, goal oriented, and look forward to a bright future. They also have a very good sense of humor. Each one starts the day eager to get going, whether it is to chop and stack wood (by hand) in anticipation of a long Maine winter, biking twenty miles, running five or more miles, teaching aerobics classes, or swimming a few laps. I want to thank them for giving me the gift of a new and positive perception of aging not as a frightening and mysterious passage but as a gift of found time with all kinds of new adventures.

A great idea stays just a great idea unless someone believes in you and takes the lead to turn the concept into reality. My editor and publisher, Garth Battista of Breakaway Books, has always believed in my ideas and puts up with my typos and creative spelling. He is a joy to work with. I also want to thank Allan Steinfeld, president of the New York Road Runners Club, for putting on the annual awards banquet night, my inspiration for the book. And a few of his NYRRC members fit my profile for this book perfectly and contributed their stories. Other friends took time from their busy schedules to recommend seniors for me to interview; they need to be thanked. Helene and Toshi, the sixty-five-and-over female runners whom I have had the honor of escorting to the New York Road Runners Club Awards Banquet for the last two years won their age divisions again, bringing home Tiffany plaques. I can only strive to be in their shoes when I reach their age. Amby Burfoot, editor of *Runner's World* magazine, also offered a few candidates and graciously agreed to write the "How To" section on starting a running program. Along the same lines, Rich Benyo of *Marathon and Beyond* magazine helped me find world-class senior runners and late bloomers Helen Klein and John Keston.

There are numerous fitness organizations for seniors, but I want to particularly thank Nancy Colarossi from the Huntsman World Senior Games in Utah for her referrals. This is a wonderful organization that promotes the thrill of competing in age-group divisions for fifty-years-of-age-and-over athletes, while also promoting lasting friendships and a healthy lifestyle through sports. The same holds true for the U.S. Masters Swimming organization, whose members can't say enough about the support and friendships they've made. Bill Volckening, editor of their *Swim* magazine, agreed to write the "How To" section on starting a swim program and his information is right on.

In researching medical and scientific data for *It's Never Too Late!*, I relied primarily on three books that I consider my bibles. Mary Pipher's *Another Country: The Emotional Terrain of Our Elders* is an excellent account of how seniors are treated —or sometimes mistreated—in this society. As a psychologist and expert on aging, Pipher was very helpful. Dr. Walter

Bortz, a leading expert in the field of health and aging, wrote the other two books. In *We Live Too Short and Die Too Long*, Bortz, a faculty member at Stanford University, dispels most of the myths about aging and replaces them with medical facts on how to age successfully. His follow-up book, *Dare to Be 100*, offers a point-by-point program for living long and enjoying life to its fullest. All three books should be required reading for anyone with aging parents or approaching that age themselves.

Throughout the interviews with these warm, generous people, who ranged in age from sixty-two to ninety-two, I kept hearing the voices of my grandparents and parents. Sadly, none of them are alive, but their spirit and zest for life while living are treasures to me. My grandfather passed away at eighty-fourand never missed his morning swim in Long Island Sound from April to November. Blessed with a singer's voice, he entertained the "old folks" at nursing homes until he died. They all succumbed to what Dr. Bortz refers to as avoidable diseases, but during their too-brief stay on earth they loved, nurtured, and educated us to their fullest capacity.

Finally, this book created many nights of deep discussion with my husband and children as to our own aging process. What will we be like in our sixties, seventies, eighties, and hopefully older years? What role will our children and future grandchildren play in our lives? Next year, when our youngest goes off to college and we face an empty nest, my husband foresees lots of travel, great restaurants, tennis, and biking together. I'll be running marathons till I can no longer make it to the starting line and always be on the lookout for the next challenge. Climbing Mount Kilimanjaro, like Rosemary Ennis just did at sixty-eight sounds like a great idea. And Elijah and Anna have promised (although it's not in writing) to be there for us when we start to forget to brush our teeth or turn off the stove. What more could I ask? Life is good.

  —Gail Waesche Kislevitz

INTRODUCTION

The idea for this book came to me while attending the New York Road Runners Club's annual awards banquet in February of 1999, a night when the young and not so young share the excitement and anticipation of wondering who will go home with the honors. It is clear that each generation admires the achievements of the others. Each generation has learned from the others, passing wisdom in both directions: the young teach the old new training methods and techniques while the old teach the young patience, tenacity, and endurance.

At my table were two women nominated for awards in their age categories, sixty-to-sixty-five and sixty-five-to-seventy, respectively. As the night progressed, the twenty-, thirty-, forty, and fifty-year-olds were (as expected) in great shape with lean, healthy physiques. Impressively fast on their feet, they accepted their Tiffany glass awards with enthusiasm. However, I was more impressed with the seventy-, eighty-, and ninety-year-olds who were competing for the awards. Their running accomplishments were as noteworthy and formidable as the younger group's but they had an added attraction, an aura about them that suggested they were receiving more than just a prize. They seemed to be celebrating not only their running merits but life as well. And there was plenty of competition in these age groups. A woman at the table behind me was up for the eighty-five-to-ninety age group award and lost. She was quite miffed and sat there kicking the table, vowing to do better next year.

As I drove two female friends home that night, each of whom had won her division, I wondered what had made the difference in their lives—what was the key that kept them active, alert, healthy, and far younger than their biological ages suggested? Why was Toshi, at seventy, breaking world records in her age division for the marathon? Why was Helene, at sixty-eight, able to run faster 10Ks than women half her age and bike seven miles to work every morning? I wanted to unlock their secrets, explore them, and share them with everyone. The most obvious explanation was that they had embraced a vigorous lifestyle at an age when others were giving up. Toshi and Helen weren't always athletes; in fact they came to it late in life, as did most of the people in this book.

Our society is aging. Everywhere you look, aging is the topic of the moment—from the bookstores to the baby boomers to the Internet. There is a website called RealAge that formulates exactly how old you are despite your biological age. There's another called Anti-aging, geared for those who are looking for a way to beat the clock.

In 1995 the first wave of baby boomers, defined as the 76 million Americans born during the first 18 years following World War II, turned fifty and will begin receiving Social Security benefits in 2010. The fastest-growing population segment is one-hundred-plus. What was once termed *old age* is now called *midlife*—the years between forty and seventy, with forty-five to sixty its core. By the year 2035 one in every four Americans will be over sixty-five, outnumbering the teenage population. The current projected life span is seventy-six, but some researchers believe it could and should be older. A study at Duke University by Kenneth Manton concluded that 1 percent of male babies born in 1975 can expect to live to 105, and females to reach 110. For some that is good news. For most the reaction is, "Who wants to live that long?" As Bette Davis said, "Getting old ain't for sissies."

There is a big difference between getting old and growing old. When Americans turn fifty, they receive an unsolicited birthday card in the mail from AARP, the American Association of Retired People. Does that card classify them as old? I know more than a few fifty-year-olds who ripped up their card, and the ones who keep it in their wallet are reluctant to use it for discounts at the movies. They don't look or act fifty, so why publicize it? Most mid-agers prefer the philosophy of Bernard Baruch, who commented, "To me, old age is always fifteen years older than I am."

We get old because we have birthdays every year. We grow old when we stop taking care of our bodies and mental health. Walter M. Bortz, M.D., an age specialist, wrote in the *Journal of the American Medical Association*, "There is no drug in current or prospective use that holds as much promise for sustained health as a lifetime program of physical exercise. If you take a master sheet of paper and record on it all the changes in the human body that are ascribed to aging—changes in the muscles, bones, brain, cholesterol, blood pressure, sleep habits, sexual performance, psychological inventory—and then compile a similar list of changes due to physical inactivity, you will note a striking similarity between the two lists. The near duplication of the lists shows that many of the bodily changes we have always ascribed to the normal aging process are in fact caused by disuse."

The people in this book are living proof of the positive affects of exercise on the aging process. Their stories are not incredible; their achievements are not unattainable. They are not super seniors. They are your neighbors, your parents, and your grandparents. They don't hold any secrets to their successful aging, don't view themselves as different. What they do share is a common lust for life and never falling into disuse. The message is slowly getting across. Visit your local Y at lunchtime and you'll have to fight the geriatric crowd into the pool. Scan a magazine rack and notice the proliferation of articles geared to older people. Join the Fifty-Plus Fitness Association or attend the Senior Olympic Games. Subscribe to the *National Masters News* and read about active seniors pursuing their sports. Check the website of the U.S. National Senior Sports Organization and see how you can get involved with a physical fitness program.

In 1967 a twenty-five-year-old Paul McCartney, along with John Lennon, wrote "Will you still need me, will you still feed me, when I'm sixty-four?" As Paul approaches sixty, he may want to change the lyrics.

—G. W. K., June 2000

IT'S NEVER TOO LATE!

THE CYCLING LIFE

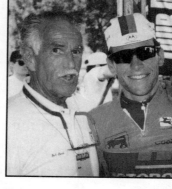

ROBERT F. BEAL

Date of birth: 10-22-27

Residence: Hingham, Massachusetts

"Coming in second means you are the first loser."
—Robert Beal

When Bob Beal was fifty-five, he decided to lose weight, quit smoking, and retire. To accomplish all these goals, he took up biking. Seventeen years later he is a competitive biker setting age-group world records and a training coach for the U.S. Cycling Federation, preparing young athletes for world class and Olympic racing. Very few people enter amateur athletics at fifty-five, but Beal took his recreational pursuits to rigorous levels of competitive achievements. Disciplined and goal oriented, Beal has had more than his share of broken bones, a fractured skull, and two heart operations. His devotion to cycling has earned him praise from many sectors. The USCF calls him a gift to cycling. His students call him inspirational, and his loving wife calls him crazy.

The second of February will be the anniversary of my second open-heart surgery. I know that date better than my wedding anniversary. Am I still going strong? At seventy-two I'm not so sure, but it doesn't stop me from putting in three hundred miles a week on my bike. To tell you the truth, getting on a bike at fifty-five for the first time in my life is probably what has kept me alive till now. I'm sure I'd be long gone if it weren't for my exercise routine these past twenty years. My memory isn't so good these days from all the times I've fallen off my bike and fractured my skull, plus being on the heart and lung machine for too long during my ten-hour surgery, but I wouldn't trade my life for anything.

Growing up in a poor family during the depression years instilled a strong work ethic in me. I've worked hard all my life, from golf caddy to checkout clerk at the grocery store. After high school I enlisted in the marines and did my stint in the war. When I returned home, I went back to work at the A&P, climbing the ladder from that checkout clerk to manager. One of the regular customers was impressed with my work and hired me to do odd jobs for him in my off hours. I built a retaining wall in his yard, saving him thousands of dollars from the contractors who were bidding on the job. In 1948 I got married and in 1950 reenlisted in the marines for a tour of duty. Back home in 1954, I resumed work at A&P. The man I built the retaining wall for remembered me and offered me a job working in an architectural engineering supply house. After working there for quite a while, two Harvard students who had a similar but smaller business came by with plans to merge and expand the business. I wasn't interested at first, but as their business grew, we became partners. Over the next twenty years we became the world leaders in our field. The company was called the Charrette Corporation.

During this time my health took a backseat to the business. Working a hundred hours a week, getting to bed at two in the morning, living on two packs of Camels a day, and getting fat was my routine. I was totally out of shape, ballooning up to

245 pounds, but would never consider wasting business hours at a doctor's office for a checkup. Even bleeding ulcers couldn't get me to change my routine and take my health seriously. But something happened at work that changed the course of my life. My Harvard partners wanted to keep expanding the business. We were already the best in the world but they wanted to also be the biggest. I thought their expansion plans were crazy. To me, being the best was more important than being the biggest. One Friday afternoon I just couldn't take the pressure anymore and walked out. Never went back.

Now that I had time to actually do things like cutting the lawn, I went to the garage to take out the lawn mower. My oldest son had just been married and received a set of bikes as a wedding gift, which they were keeping in my garage. It was my good fortune that these bikes were blocking the lawn mower. Already thinking of getting in shape, I hopped on the bike—although I was secretly telling myself I was crazy for even trying to ride it. I wobbled down the street for three miles just like a kid trying to ride without training wheels for the first time. The next day I thought I'd die from the pain. It was awful, but it gave me a challenge. This could be fun, I told myself. This could be my new exercise. I started to ride more and bought my own bike. Six months later I entered my first training race, thirty-two miles. I honestly didn't know what I was getting myself into and couldn't even finish the race. I got blown away. Not wanting to admit defeat, I decided the problem was the bike, not me, so I went out and bought a thousand-dollar bike. I didn't do any better at my next race and I began to realize I didn't need a better bike, I needed a better body. It is the engine, not the machine that makes for good performance and I was a poor engine.

By now I had quit smoking. Just threw the packs away and never picked up another cigarette. To this day I still get the craving to smoke, but I haven't since the day I tossed the packs. I knew I had to get serious about biking if I wanted to race so I joined a bike club and started training. The support was just what I needed. At the time I remember talking to the "older guys"—and now I'm one of them. They taught me about pacing and cadence and other things about biking you can only learn from the experience of the experts. My son and his friends also offered encouragement, which meant a lot to me. I live for my kids, and I was finally doing something we could share. The camaraderie was wonderful and it still is one of the biggest reasons I've stayed in biking. I have never met such nice people before. The competitors, spectators and officials are all top-notch people and I don't think I could have done it without their enthusiasm.

When I finally won my first medal, it was thrilling. It was a thirty-five-mile race, and there were lots of people in my age group, fifty-five to sixty. Actually, there is always a well-stocked group in my age division at the races. Before I started racing, I was more than a little uncomfortable with the whole idea. What am I doing out here? I'm fifty-five years old, fat and out of shape. I don't belong here. But in my first year of biking I competed in twenty-two races.

When I was sixty-two I entered the New England Championships and expected to win. Instead I just barely finished and really felt bad about that. Not only emotionally but physically as well. I was spent after the race. In those days, before heart monitors, we checked our endurance levels by using what was called a resting pulse. For a good athlete, a normal resting pulse was forty. Mine was usually down to thirty-eight if I was racing well. That day, my resting pulse was thirty-two. Being naïve about such things, I didn't realize that was the first sign something was terribly wrong. My pulse continued to drop to twenty-eight, to twenty, and by the third day I went to my doctor, who took an EKG and rushed me to the hospital for a pacemaker. Luckily for me, my doctor was also a cyclist and advised me to get right back on the bike, as it was good exercise. Later that same year, 1989, I was racing up a hill and fell off the bike. It was actually a heart attack, but I didn't take notice of it. In fact, I got right back on. The next day I entered another race at White River Junction. I needed to take at least third place to win the overall Masters championships, which I did. But I came home feeling absolutely terrible. The next day I had a triple bypass to correct what the doctors said was total heart block. But I'm not a quitter and was racing again in less than three months. During recovery I walked a little bit each day. The pain was terrible but I wanted to get back on that bike as fast as I could. It hurt just to sneeze or cough. The only problem I had when I could finally ride again was getting used to that hard seat all over again.

My wife of fifty-two years thinks I'm nuts. But I keep telling her and my friends that if it weren't for the biking, I'd already be dead. Through biking, I've quit smoking, have an outlet for stress, changed my diet from steak and junk food to egg whites, fruits, and vegetables, and also monitor my portions. Growing up poor, whenever we did have food on the plate we ate every morsel, because food was not meant to be wasted. That fact always stayed with me. Even when things got better I ate large quantities and always scraped my plate clean. Now I've had to adjust that, and I only eat what I need. My heart problems were due to blockage and God knows what else. My favorite way to explain the fact that I am still around is that I am in great shape for the shape I'm in.

My racing started to get longer in distance and better in performance. I got interested in cyclocross, which takes place during fall and winter. It requires riding on skinny tires in less-than-ideal conditions which could include snow, sleet, and severe windchill. At times we have to get off our bikes and carry them across streams or other terrain too rough for them. It's very exciting and instead of hanging up my bike for the official off season I can continue to ride and stay trained while maintaining cardiovascular fitness.

During this time, I was thinking of becoming a coach so I could give something back to the sport I love so much. I was asked by the U.S. Cycling Federation to come out to Colorado and consider coaching prospective Olympians. That was just what I was looking for, and after intensive training I received my coaching certificate. Since then, I have continued my coaching credentials to become an elite trainer and coach, massage therapist, strength and conditioning coach, personal trainer, and *soigneur.* That last term sounds fancy but it means that I take total care of the athletes. I am their massage therapist, prepare their food, and look after their general well-being. I'm also responsible for everyone's bike and gear when we travel. You cannot begin to imagine the logistics of taking a team overseas. All the riders have at least two bikes, all their gear, and all the technical equipment, massage tables—it's endless. And I'm the guy who has to get it all there all accounted for. That's what *soigneur* means.

My coaching responsibilities have been very rewarding. I headed the Junior Olympic training camp in Colorado and one year a very talented kid came to us, and I just knew he was special. I took him under my wing and helped him reach his potential. That kid, Lance Armstrong, went on to win the World Championship Road Race in 1992 and won the Tour de France in 1999, the second American to ever win and the first American to win on an American team. Armstrong's victory was twofold, having beaten testicular cancer just three years prior to the more-than-two-thousand-mile race. He is my pride and joy, and my favorite biking possessions are his bright yellow biking jerseys that he has autographed for me. I am always on the lookout for another Armstrong, although they don't come by that often.

My coaching responsibilities have taken me to Poland, England, Denmark, Russia, Cuba, Slovakia, the Czech Republic and other interesting places. While some locations may sound exotic, others have been less than ideal. In Guatemala, for instance, a race that was under way was never completed because two political factions began shooting at each other on the course. There has also been a much greater emphasis on drugs and drug testing in the past ten years. Immediately after a race, the first three finishers are escorted from their bikes and tested. The other thing we have to worry about on the course is drug sabotage. The sabotage occurs by offering competitors drinks along the course that are laced with an illegal substance, which will test positive for drugs when the rider finishes the race. I only allow my team to accept drinks from their own teammates.

My trials and travails on my own race circuit continued to plague me. Four years ago I was on a downhill doing fifty-five miles per hour around a curve and lost control. I broke thirty-eight bones, including my neck, and had to be helicoptered out in a gurney from the gully where I landed. The funny thing was, my bike was fine! Three weeks prior to that injury, I was blindsided by a truck that ran a red light. My helmet saved me in that instance. A good biker usually obeys the street laws; it's the cars that don't. In 1999 I had my second open-heart surgery on February 2. The blockage had built up and I started to get angina pains. I couldn't even walk a half mile without pain running right down the middle of my chest. But believe it or not, I could bike all I wanted except for hills. Never felt pain while biking, although my endurance was way down. The operation was terrible. While being prepped I went into total cardiac arrest. After they brought me back to normal, the doctors had to enter my chest from under my armpit because of the scar tissue buildup from the first surgery, breaking my ribs along the way. The operation took ten hours and the recovery time was also ten times worse than the first operation. Everything hurt, including my legs because they took veins from my leg to replace the blocked arteries. My first steps were slow; building up to a walk, and it took four months before I could get back on a bike. The worse part was gaining twenty pounds. Weight is the biggest scourge for a biker, so I was very upset with myself.

I always have to do my best. My training includes biking three hundred miles a week and daily workouts at the gym. I get up at 4 A.M. to get to the gym where I train others as well as myself and then start biking at 8:30 for two or three hours. I've already put in fifty miles before I pick up the morning paper and bring it home to my wife. She doesn't go to my races anymore, because she doesn't like to see me crash. Sometimes I go out again in the afternoon. I love it, despite the constant pain I'm usually experiencing. My overall medication involves taking twenty pills a day, some of which help to relieve the pain. But riding my bike is my real therapy. I also have some new form of arthritis. My joints are a mess but there's no sense complaining. I know there are many people who think I'm crazy, but I don't bother to explain myself to anyone. During the winter months I do mountain biking in the woods, which is wonderful. I go slower so I get to see the snowcapped trees, animals, and pretty winter landscapes.

One of the side benefits for me of all my injuries and accidents is learning how to use the computer. I suffer from short-memory loss due to all my skull injuries and having been too long on the respirator during my second ten-hour operation. It was really bothering me that I couldn't remember things, so I started keeping files on the computer so I would have some kind of recall. It also helps to work my mind, almost like a mental exercise to help the circuits stay alert. I actually coach over the computer now. I'm working with many bikers who send me their workouts and their times and I adjust them every week and send them back a new workout.

I worked hard my whole life and now I am still working hard but enjoying it more. I've also been blessed with an understanding and loving wife, four wonderful children and six grandchildren. They give me reason to live. I've trained and coached all over the United States and overseas. It is what I do. I can't stay away from my bike. The mental aspects of biking are very rewarding. It teaches you discipline and moderation, the main keys to enjoying biking. Going into a world-class sporting profession at such a late time in my life is perhaps proof that if you want something bad enough, it's never too late.

THE UNSINKABLE IVY BROWNE

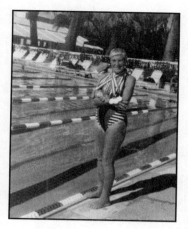

IVY BROWNE

Date of birth 1-8-15

Residence: Reno, Nevada

"Create a life that is burning every moment."
—T. S. Eliot

When I first phoned Ivy Browne, the voice that answered was so youthful sounding that I was tempted to ask to speak with her mother. But it was Ivy, full of vigor at seven in the morning. We talked for a while and then she cut me short, saying, "Darlin' I'd love to chat some more but I am late for an exercise class, and I'm the instructor. Call me back later." She had been up since 5:30.

There is one characteristic regarding a healthy aging process that all the experts agree on: attitude. A positive outlook on life makes a world of difference. A positive attitude creates an atmosphere that encourages effort. Ivy's attitude seems to say, "Don't invite old age into the house." She thinks she's forty, not eighty-five. And with her schedule and energy, who's going to defy her? She shoots from the hip and if you don't like what she has to say, don't listen.

As a kid I was always standing on my head, flippin' around and on the go. I was a red-haired, freckle faced tomboy. If times were different I would have received an athletic scholarship, but not back then so I didn't even go to college. Today, at eighty-five, nothing has changed much. I'm still on the go all the time, red haired and freckled. My ancestors were Findlanders and to those roots I credit my energy and staying power. In fact, I have to go to the hospital next week because I keep wearing out my pacemaker.

When I was nineteen I swam across the San Francisco Bay on a dare. It was more than five miles and took me two hours and six minutes. That record was just broken by another female three years ago, by just four minutes. I feel pretty good about that, considering she had access to tidal charts and other information that I never used. But after swimming the bay, I contracted typhoid fever and didn't swim or do any form of exercise for forty-eight years. From the age of nineteen to sixty-eight, I never swam a stroke.

Married for the first time at twenty-three, the relationship lasted ten years. My second marriage lasted four years; my third lasted ten years, and my fourth lasted three years. Some people collect butterflies, I collected husbands. The marriages weren't that bad, I just gave up everything for my husbands and never did learn that that's not the way to keep a marriage. I was a good wife; did the shopping, cooking, and cleaning. Everything they wanted was handed to them on a platter. Worked hard at it. My husbands always had a home cooked meal on the table when they returned from work. I spoiled then so badly they stopped contributing to the marriage and let me do all the work. Then I'd tire of it and just up and leave. But I never did learn my lesson. One husband was a golfer and I would get up early with him, go to the golf course, and sit in the car waiting for eight hours. Oh, every once in a while I'd get up and go for a walk or read the paper, but I waited for him. That's the kind of wife I was. The best thing about my marriages was the birth of my son, with my first husband. After having typhoid, it took me three years to get pregnant. My doctor didn't believe me when I said I wanted to get pregnant but I did. And in the timeframe I predicted. Told my doctor it would take three years and it did.

In 1943 I moved from Oakland to Tahoe and worked my butt off. Did all kinds of odd jobs like shoveling snow, housekeeping, and catering parties. You don't know snow till you've spent a winter in Tahoe. Because it was a seasonal place, I had to earn enough money in four months to last twelve. My cleaning motto was, "Not one grain of sand in the house." I had the same customer for thirty-nine years, so I know I was good. The parties were hard work, too. All the celebrities came to Tahoe over the holidays and I was working day and night hosting parties. There was never any time for myself, or for exercise. But my work was so demanding and so physical, I was always in good shape; strong and healthy. On the other hand, my son suffered terribly from allergies. He was in and out of so many hospitals; I had to work two or three jobs just to pay the bills. The one problem with walking out on all my husbands was not getting any alimony. The doctors never did find the right medicine or cure for him, so I started researching his symptoms myself and learned about food allergies. Started preparing special meals for him. That was the only thing that kept him off the death list. Not the doctors, me. Whatever I did back then for him worked. Now he is healthy and married, and I am a grandmother three times over and have a great-granddaughter.

The years I lived in Tahoe were very isolating for us. After twenty years I'd had enough and moved to Reno. Not know-

ing anyone, I decided to join a swim club. The first day I dove
in the pool and just swam like a fish, not even thinking that
forty-eight years had passed by since I last swam. I was swimming so fast the guard asked if he could time me. He told me
of a masters swim meet coming up, but I didn't even know
what he was talking about. Tahoe does that to you; you forget
there's a world outside. Anyhow, I wasn't interested in any
form of competition. But the next day when I went back, I
got kind of curious. He timed me for the mile and afterward I
wasn't even breathing hard. He told me I was close to breaking the masters record for the mile. Now, that got my attention! I entered that swim meet and at seventy-six years of age
broke the Pacific Coast record for my age division.

After I discovered the Senior Olympics and the Huntsman
World Games in Utah, I started doing everything: the shot
put, javelin, discus, and basketball. You name it, I do it. But
swimming is the easiest for me, although I never train or
practice for anything. Who has time to train? And who has a
javelin or discus lying around the garage? During the summer of 1990 I set a world record that still holds for a 10K
swim, which is 6.2 miles. No breaks, just straight swimming.
Took me four hours and nineteen minutes. At one time they
just about forced me to stop and drink some apple juice, but it
was so darn sweet I threw up.

I think my endurance comes from always swimming in
open waters when I was a kid. Once you learn to swim in the
ocean, you can swim anywhere. I still do the Waikiki three-
mile open-ocean swim. I'm usually the oldest woman so I
always come home with at least two trophies. The last time I
did it, a bunch of us nearly drowned. We started the race in
hurricane winds. One hundred people dropped out at the

start, but not me. I was managing pretty well until about three hundred yards from the end, when a group of us got caught in a whirlpool. The force kept twirling me around and around for what seemed like hours. I just remembered to keep looking up, looking for a patch of blue sky to make sure I was alive and facing in the right direction. When I was dragged down, the coral scratched my eyes. At one point I lost my sixty-five-dollar goggles, but they were so damned expensive I went looking for them and by golly found them. One of the volunteers came out on a surfboard to try to rescue us but she was having such a hard time, I thought I'd be better on my own. The whirlpool finally died down enough for us to get back to shore, which was the end of the race so I eventually finished. I do these events for fun. I really don't care about winning. I came on the masters scene so fast and out of nowhere, and with such a winning streak, that some of the regulars who were used to winning would cry when they saw me. They'd say, "I used to win before you showed up." I was ready to quit because I didn't want to make them cry. I just enjoy being out there. I beat them. They beat me. Who cares?

Moving to Reno didn't mean retirement for me. I still work and even drive back to Tahoe one day a week to clean house. It's 105 miles round trip, but it's good money and I like the clients. I need a new car, though, and went car shopping the other day. Most dealers don't want to sell a car to an eighty-five-year-old woman, but I always manage to convince them in the end. I also use the car for my volunteer work at the Gospel Mission in downtown Reno on Thursdays, delivering bread to the poor. I've been doing this for twenty years. Fifty loaves of bread every week. Then I have to drive to Utah for the Huntsman Games, which is a fourteen-hour drive. For that I do force myself to stop every hundred miles or so and get out for a stretch and walk around the car a few times. I like to keep busy. If you don't move, you rust. Then there's my aerobics class; I'm the instructor. I teach an early-morning class and I have to say I am a tough instructor. I also teach aquacize, tai chi, yoga, and give massages. My group is called Super Seniors.

In 1996 I was fitted for pacemaker. I started to get dizzy spells and went to see a doctor, who wanted to take an EKG, but I was already scheduled at a swim meet in Kentucky so postponed the test. At the swim meet I started getting dizzy again but kept swimming no matter how dizzy I got. Besides, I was on my way to a gold medal. Luck was on my side and a doctor was at the meet. When the dizziness got worse, he called an ambulance. I have never been so embarrassed as when they carried me out of the pool on a gurney. But you better believe I was clutching my gold medal as they wheeled me away. My heart was fibrillating and just tuckered out so I got a pacemaker. They wanted to operate then and there but I had a plane ticket back home and couldn't afford to change it so I flew home and had the operation in Reno.

I get tested every week to ensure that the pacemaker batteries are still working. At my age, combined with my level of activity, the doctors are never sure how long the batteries will last. Actually I am a good patient. I never lie, never complain and always follow their instructions. If they tell me to take it easy for a day or two, I do. We get along very well. One time at my regular exam, the doctors noticed the wires that attach the pacemaker to my arm were broken. They fixed it, but I was scheduled for a meet the next day so I swam with only one arm. It's tough doing the butterfly stroke with one arm! In fact I did all the strokes with only one arm. Executed a perfect dive, backstroke, breaststroke, you name it. The event had to go on. It was very funny. Everyone was betting whether I'd make it to the other side. But you'd better bet I did. I've also had a total hip replacement, which was a nuisance because I had to teach my classes on crutches for a while, as well as shoulder and knee surgeries, but you wouldn't know it. I let the pain get to the point where I can't stand it any longer before I let a doctor take over. Things hurt. So what. A lot of people like to sit around moaning and groaning about what hurts, but if they just got up and did something they wouldn't have time to think about that stuff. We all need a push, a kick in the pants, and for me it's swimming. I can't sit around thinking about all the places on my body that hurt. It's a waste of time.

I also keep busy by volunteering at hospitals as a guinea pig. Basically, I feel I am helping others by donating my time and body to science. This past year I volunteered on a survey for cancer, one for rheumatism and one for rheumatoid arthritis. Each survey takes about six months. I get a nice certificate at the end and the knowledge that I've helped science help others.

I'm not ready to slow down yet. My life is full with lots of friends, an active social life, and too many parties to attend. You could say I'm on top of the world, or at least the top of my eighty-plus age group for competition. Still love men, but have no steadies. I don't want to get into a long-term relationship because they just die off. Men die off fast. They get one symptom and go *per-clunk* and it's over. I'd have to date someone thirty-five to keep up with me.

My philosophy is: "Be happy." Why not? I don't like to think of the alternative. I don't have arthritis, don't wear glasses, haven't any memory loss or signs of cancer. Don't eat much red meat or starches; I'm not big on sandwiches. When people ask me my philosophy for life, I tell them it is very simple: "Live a good clean life with lots of enthusiasm and energy." That's my prescription. I'm going to live to the day I die.

My biggest bugaboo right now is not being able to find a sponsor to help defray the cost of my travel and lodging when I go to my sports events. I've called all the airlines but they won't sponsor me. Heck, you'd think someone would want to help an old lady get to the Senior Olympics! The expenses have actually made me slow down. I am only participating in events that I can drive to. But I'll keep going no matter. Don't want to rust.

THE TRI-ING NUN

SISTER MADONNA BUDER

Date of birth: 7-24-30

Residence: Spokane, Washington

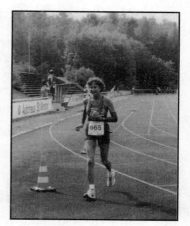

"Never let yesterday use up today." —Richard Nelson

I spent months tracking down Sister Buder after her name came up a few times as someone I should interview. When I finally got in touch, she was surprised I had gone to such lengths to find her. She doesn't think of herself as a celebrity, just someone with God-given talents who wants to dedicate those talents to helping others. After she ran her first marathon at fifty-two, exercise redirected her life, and she has gone on to compete in over two hundred triathlons, including thirteen Hawaiian Ironman events, nine Canadian Ironman events, and two in New Zealand. She was selected as the female Grandmaster Triathlete of the Year in San Diego in February 2000. Along the way she has suffered serious injuries, but through her prayer, devotion, and determination, she always manages to find her way back on course.

People always ask me how I am able to compete in the Ironman competitions at my age and do so well. I have a very simple answer: I don't know. But I do think I owe some of it to the strong genes I inherited from my dad. He was a champion oarsman. My mother, who considered herself an oarsman's widow, finally got to spend time with him after the boathouse burned down. She was very creative and spiritual by nature, which balanced his practicality and physical prowess. Maybe that's what led me to the convent. I attended public school up until sixth grade and had a grand old time. I didn't learn much except through osmosis and the girl-boy parties resulting in kissing games. Once my mother found out about my extracurricular activities, that was it for me. I was sent to Catholic school and reality set in fast. I was far behind in subject matter, so one of the nuns took me under her wing. She was very loving and nurturing and tutored me on the side. She was a big influence on my decision to enter the convent, which I did at the age of twenty-three.

In 1978 I was attending a workshop on the Oregon coast. One of the priests was expounding on the virtues of running. He made it sound like a cure for everything, that we should all take it up. I wasn't a runner, although I had always enjoyed interactive sports and showing horses. I couldn't understand the concept of just running for no good reason. I needed a goal. The priest suggested to me that people make their own goals; that something as simple as running between the jetties on the beach could be a goal. Later on that day, I slipped on a pair of secondhand sneakers that had been given to me and ran between the jetties. The distance was about half a mile and I did it in just about five minutes. Never having run before, I didn't know that that was considered a good time. The priest was on the deck when I came up from the beach and asked me about my run. He told me if I could do that, I should keep running, because God had given me a talent. I continued running between the jetties for the remainder of the week.

Back home, I decided to use the ball field behind the gym for running. Seven times around the field was approximately a mile, so that became my daily run. A few weeks later I saw an advertisement for an 8.2-mile race—a big event called the Bloomsday Race, which was to take place in a month or so. The thought of all those people herded together repulsed me. It was hard enough to run without elbowing your way through a crowd. This was the second year of the run and it boasted over five thousand participants. That night I received a call from my mother with news that one of my brothers was going through a difficult time. Right then and there I decided to do the run for my brother. When I explained this to Mother, she was quite dismayed and tried to talk me out of it, but I had made up my mind. She called me back a few days later and said my brother, who had run track in high school, didn't think I should be doing it. They were concerned that I would get injured running 8.2 miles with very little experience. But I had a goal; I wanted the Lord to take my will to endure the race and transfer that will to my brother to get through his difficulty . I was forty-nine years old but was determined.

After four weeks of training I finally worked up to four miles, but I was miserable. Coughing, sneezing, spasms, hurting. I thought it was the pollen I was stirring up, so I switched to running on the streets but that was worse. My knees swelled, my calves tightened up, my ankles hurt, and my feet had blisters. My entire body was going through the way of the cross. With one week to go before the race, I just didn't know how I was going to get through it. I started sobbing, thinking I would have to give up this quest. When I ceased sobbing, I received an interior message. The Lord was saying, "In my agony in the garden I did not know how many people down through the ages would respond to my act of love either. I also had to step out in faith." My response was, "Okay Lord, I can't do this, so you will have to be my strength." Having said this, I dragged myself to the door and went for a run regardless of my condition. I didn't feel any better but I didn't feel any worse either. How could I? There was nothing else left to hurt! I was so naïve about the art of running. Still in my hand-me-down tennis shoes, I wasn't stretching, warming up, cooling down, drinking water— nothing that would have spared me all that agony. Finally, one of our order's benefactors heard of my training and offered to buy me running shoes. I felt somewhat guilty spending thirteen dollars of his money for a pair of scruffy-looking running shoes, especially since I never planned to wear them again. The last thing I did wrong was to break in the new shoes so shortly before the race that they ended up breaking me instead, with blisters.

The day of the event was a beautiful, cloudless May morning, like the morning of the Resurrection. My plan was to run for two miles, walk four minutes, run two miles, and so forth, but of course I forgot to wear a watch. I was toward the rear of the pack and the camaraderie was wonderful. That's where all the fun is! When I got to the finish, I went down to the Spokane River and waded in the cold water to help heal my legs. I had not planned on doing this, but when I saw the water somehow I knew it would it soothe my throbbing muscles. I truly think it is this survival instinct that has allowed me to survive all the subsequent years of competitions.

Despite all the hardships and pains of running the race, I placed fourth in my age group. At the finish line, flyers were being passed out for another local race. What the heck; I already had the shoes and I never wanted to put my body through this again, so perhaps I needed to just keep going.

After steadily running one race a month, two years later I decided to tackle a marathon. Why not? I thought it'd be a great goal to run a marathon in my fifties. As I was preparing for my first marathon, I also decided to set a goal to qualify for the Boston Marathon, with a finishing time of 3:30 or less. At fifty-two, I didn't know how I was going to do that but finished with twelve seconds remaining. Now that I'd qualified, I needed permission from my order to travel to Boston. Afraid they wouldn't support me, I went straight to the bishop. Apprehensively, I approached him with my story, adding that I wanted to do this for a cause greater than myself by collecting funds for multiple sclerosis. After taking pains to explain to him that I did not want to cause a scandal or attract an unwanted media blitz for the order, he sat back with a droll grin and finally said, "Sister, I just wish some of my priests would do what you're doing."

I ran Boston wearing a T-shirt the nuns had given me paraphrasing a quote from St. Paul about racing toward the goal. I think I was the first nun to ever run Boston. And once again, I ran naïve. The last time I'd eaten was 6:30 A.M., and the race didn't begin until noon. I was aware of being hungry before the race even began. By mile twenty-four my legs had turned to lead. I couldn't lift them. I was afraid I'd have to walk. It became the way of the cross for me, as the crowds moved on us during the last two miles. It was suffocating. Somehow my faith pulled me through and I finished in 3:32. Having raised four thousand dollars in pledges for MS, I went back the next year to do the same again.

The next big event I tackled was a half Ironman triathlon (1.2-mile swim, 56-mile bike ride, and 13.1-mile run). More foolishness. At first I outright rejected the idea, but it wouldn't let go of me because now I knew I could run, and I wasn't afraid of the water. I was pretty sure I could complete it, so I gave in to the quest. And once again, I did it all wrong. Graduating from a balloon-tire bike to a ten-speed bike was bad enough. Swimming 1.2 miles wasn't so bad, but after the 56-mile bike ride with strong headwinds, my legs were trashed and I still had to run 13 miles. It seems I always do things the hard way. But once again, when I finished I wanted more. Learning from my mistakes, I decided to tackle a full Ironman distance (2.4-mile swim, 112-mile bike, and 26.2-mile run). For me, it's the challenge; it's there to be done, so why not try? Of course, I have to have a certain amount of faith that I can pull it off. To that end, I am determined never to give in. I will exert every fiber in my body to finish once I am committed to a race. It's not a fitness thing; it's a spiritual quest. God gave me these talents, and I want to return the glory to him by doing my utmost. The Hawaiian Ironman symbolized my eternal goal. More than anything else, it was a spiritual propulsion that impelled me to enter this most difficult challenge. The other reason I enjoy events such as these is that they take place outdoors and I love nature. The largeness of the great outdoors has a way of making us realize how small we really are in this big pond and that the problems we carry around with us are not as overwhelming as we make them. Nothing is too big to handle; everything can be solved. God is everywhere in nature, and observing nature can help us solve our problems if we just let him.

I started to prepare for the 1985 Hawaiian Ironman, three major setbacks kept me from competing that year. Most of them had to do with injuries from bike accidents while training. I've come to resemble a fragile Dresden china doll that has nicks and chips in every place imaginable. My first major injury was in 1984 while training in St. Louis. I was using a borrowed bike and was not familiar with the "suicide" brakes on the handlebars; nor was I wearing a helmet. For some reason I had to brake fast and went flying over the handlebar. I landed just an inch from striking my head on the curb. Behind me was a huge city bus. The driver had stopped to let out a passenger, who came running over to help. I thought I was fine, but that was due to the shock. Someone offered to take me to the emergency room, but I kept protesting. All I wanted was a ride home. Reluctantly I was taken home and it was only then that I realized something was wrong, when I saw the blood on the white bathroom tiles. I ended up in the hospital with a compound fractured elbow, fractured jaw, dislocated scapular, and multiple abrasions. As I lay in bed swathed in bandages, all I could talk about was my race and the Ironman and when I could start training again. The doctor shook his head and said, 'Healing is a matter of time. You can't rush it. You must give your body a chance to heal itself. Put aside these plans for the Ironman.' But I couldn't. I'd slip out of bed unobserved and run up and down the stairwell so my legs wouldn't atrophy. When I was discovered, they discharged me sooner than intended. The doctor warned me that even a slight bump would damage the healing process. I was determined to continue my training and a few weeks later ran the Diet Pepsi 10K Championships in New York with my arm in a sling and a sign on my back that read, INJURED RUNNER. NO PASSING ON THE RIGHT, PLEASE. I persevered to the end, finishing fourth in my age group against national competition.

After the accident, the hardest thing to do was get back on the bike. Psychologically, I needed to prove to myself that I could still ride the Ironman just three months away. In August my spirits were lifted when I successfully completed a half Ironman triathlon. But then came September! I was riding my bike back to the convent in heavy traffic after a training ride. It was rush hour, and as I tried to cross the four lanes of traffic, the light changed. A car came from behind and was not going to stop. I had to swerve to avoid a collision and went down hard. My hip was broken in two places. I remember looking up to heaven and saying, "Lord, what do you have against me doing the Ironman?"

The two-and-a-half-hour surgery was a success. I came out with extra adornments: a screw in the femur and a plate with five pins along the shank. The transition from wheelchair to walker to crutches took longer than anticipated due to my contracting phlebitis. I limped for four years.

The following November, just as I was getting my life back on track, my father died of a heart attack. Now more than ever, I needed direction in life and I was determined to do the Ironman the following October. I concentrated on my training and everything was finally falling into place. However, with only six weeks to go, I was on a training ride in Australia and got hit by a car. I ended up with broken ribs and a chipped heel, but continued training and flew on to Hawaii. The night before the event, the race director announced that we might be getting a hurricane, but not to worry—the race would go on no matter what. The next day we started the 2.4-mile swim in two-to-four-foot ocean swells. My ribs were still sore, and the extra battering didn't help. The currents were too intense for me and I found myself swimming in place, unable to make any headway the last fifty yards. Missing the cutoff time by four minutes, I was disqualified. I dried off, got something to eat, and then decided to ride the bike course anyway. I didn't do it as a participant, but I was there, so why not try it? Well, I think the Lord wanted me to do that because I ended up coaxing a minister who was in last place and desperately needed some encouragement to pull him along. I acted as his carrot. With only seconds to spare, he rolled in to the bike finish. Since it was getting dark, I left him on his own for the run, calling out "Go for God, Padre," words he had emblazoned on his handlebars. He was the very last official finisher of the competition, and God and I got him through.

The next year, 1986, was a good year for me, and I finally made it through the Hawaiian Ironman after winning the New Zealand Ironman seven months earlier. Having already done the swimming and biking the year before, I knew I could get through it, since running was my forte. I was pleased to have competed that year and to have earned second place.

Truly, there are times when I can't understand myself why I do this. I've gone on to complete the Hawaiian Ironman thirteen times, the Canadian Ironman nine times, and the New Zealand Ironman twice. I've set records in two age divisions in both the Canadian and Hawaiian Ironman. This year I'll turn seventy and I am looking forward to setting another record in these two events. I know my records will be broken someday; I just can't understand why it has taken so long. There are people out there capable of doing it; they just don't realize it yet.

Exercise has redirected my life. I never dreamed I'd be the triathlon nun. It all boils down to an element of faith, belief in yourself, and belief in the God who made you. One night before a race the skies opened up with wind, lightning, and a full-force rain. At the prerace dinner the participants wondered if the race would be canceled. The race director asked me to say a prayer. The right words flowed forth and seemed to put everyone at ease. I reminded them that God loves us and was not going to let anything happen to us that would be self-destructive. With a collective faith we can relax in mind and spirit, taking what he gives us with trust and courage. The next day was perfect!

My life has been full and varied but not without its trials. Always, my faith carries me through. Maybe I am destined for a long life to help and inspire others. I've dedicated each leg of the triathlon to each of my three brothers and their respective needs. I've helped to raise money for diabetes, heart disease, MS—you name the illness and I've run for it. I've used my skills as a photographer to create inspirational slide presentations. I've advocated for troubled juveniles. I've written two books, *I Have Finished the Race* and *The Man Behind the Miracles*, and donated the proceeds to worthy causes.

Even though I feel fulfilled by using the talents God gave me, it seems there is always more to do. Life is never at a standstill, and neither am I. This reminds me of the quote from St. Augustine: "We are restless, oh Lord, until we rest in thee."

SKATING KEEPS HIM IN LINE

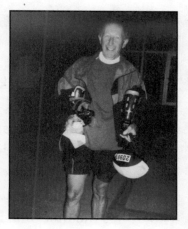

AL CHECHIK

Date of birth: 10-13-34

Residence: Bayfield, Wisconsin

"There is no cure for birth and death, save to enjoy the interval." —George Santayana

Al's story of loss and survival deeply affected me, as it will most likely affect everyone. Al had to learn to live his life without his wife, Margaret. He instinctively knew that exercise would play a role in his healing process. When they were married in 1985, they had exchanged watches instead of rings, explaining that "the only thing you have together is time." Al has learned to put his time to good use, helping others understand and travel through the grieving process.

Upon retiring from my corporate day job in June 1996, my wife and I prepared to open the bed-and-breakfast we had been planning for some six years in northern Wisconsin, on the edge of Lake Superior. Margaret and I had been married for eleven years, and we were both looking forward to this new retired life. In preparation, we had worked together in the planning, decorating, advertising, and business aspects of the B&B. We greeted our first guests on June 14, 1996. Less than six weeks later, Margaret was diagnosed with inoperable stomach cancer. She passed away on October 20, at age forty-nine.

I decided to continue with the B&B, since it was something we shared, and I knew she would want me to go on. Margaret was also part of the reason I decided to enter my first in-line skating marathon in 1997. During that first year after her death, I did a lot of thinking about my life alone. Among other necessary changes, skating a marathon seemed a good way to pick up a challenge, to have a goal. At sixty-two, it was the first time I had ever entered such an event.

Backing up a bit: I had spent most of my life in Wisconsin, employed in the communications field for thirty-seven years. In high school I enjoyed playing all sports, but never competed at the varsity level. After college I tried to stay active with a few sports—tennis, golf, basketball, softball. I was married (for the first time) in 1959 and found that work and raising a family took priority over everything else. So I suffered the sins of neglect, and even though I stayed in reasonable shape, I realized the need to tone. In my late forties I took up running for a while, but wasn't what you'd call a natural runner and never considered running a marathon. Margaret and I ran together occasionally, but neither of us really had a passion for it. Then, when I was fifty-five, Margaret's nephew from New York came to visit during the summer and brought his Rollerblades. I had never seen inline skating up close and became interested. I borrowed his skates and found that I liked it. A few days later I bought my own pair, and that was all it took. I started skating regularly—just for fun, no thought about competing. At the time Margaret and I lived in a condo in Madison, Wisconsin, and nearby was a new business park with plenty of smooth, lightly traveled roads. That's where I headed several times a week during spring, summer, and fall. Eventually, I started to take my skates along on business trips and always tried to squeeze in a few miles, often in downtown areas that were quite deserted after 6 P.M., or around 6 A.M.

When Margaret and I moved to Bayfield, a town of less than seven hundred people, we found it wasn't an area conducive to skating. Rural and quite hilly, with few smooth roads. The spring of 1996 there was no time for skating anyway; first the opening of the B&B, then Margaret's illness, which consumed us during the summer and fall. It was the spring of 1997, six months after her death, before I even thought about getting back to skating. I found a few decent country roads, and eventually discovered Madeline Island, a twenty-minute ferry ride from Bayfield. For longer workouts it was the best, with flat, fairly deserted roads and a state park only six miles from the ferry dock, so I could skate along quiet country roads with views of Lake Superior and get in six to ten miles (plus an ice cream cone) before heading back to the ferry.

Physically, skating was much easier on my legs and knees than running was. My personal goal wasn't to build muscle, become stronger, or keep going farther; it was to stay active and have fun in the process. I was familiar with the positive aspects of exercise, but, having known a few runners, I refused to become obsessed with the need for a schedule—to go x miles in x minutes x times a week. I just wanted to have that good feeling of moving along through the countryside and enjoying myself. As a bonus, I found myself in better mental shape. Skating is a good way to get exercise if you move with some degree of speed. You don't have to punish your body to get results. And I like the feeling of freedom, whether I'm skating in a rural area or a city setting. I found the Chicago and Milwaukee lakeshores, the interconnected Minneapolis lakes, and downtown Green Bay especially good places to skate. You really become one with your surroundings.

Over my ten years of skating, I've added a few scars but have had only one serious accident. It happened the day of the Oklahoma City bombing. I was skating on a familiar path in Madison and came upon a new construction site. The road seemed to continue, but there was a yellow warning tape across the path. I ducked under the tape and continued. Moments later I was confronted with another tape covering metal wires that stretched across the path. It was too late to stop; I simply hit the pavement. I felt my skates jam into my sides and had the wind knocked out of me. As I lay there, a police officer patrolling the area stopped and asked if I needed help. I declined, thinking I was okay, and I started to skate home, which was about two miles away. I quickly discovered that the pain was intense, and I was bleeding from some minor cuts. I also realized I couldn't breathe without feeling a sharp pain in my chest. Bottom line: I ended up in the hospital with three fractured ribs. It was six weeks before I could even think about skating. Needless to say, that accident made me a more cautious skater.

In the period after Margaret's death, I began examining life without her. All our plans had been made together—a togetherness that no longer existed. It was time to seek new activities that I could enjoy alone. One day in June 1997, I read in the Duluth newspaper that the Northshore Inline

Marathon—the largest in-line event in the nation—would be held in mid-September. It would go from Two Harbors to Duluth, the same course used for the well known Grandma's Marathon each June. I had never heard of the event, but decided to give it a try. I blocked out the dates on my room reservation calendar so I'd have no guests on that Friday evening in September, and sent in my reservation form and check to make it official. I now had a goal that gave me a focus beyond the routine of the B&B.

The hardest part of the three months of preparation was finding a road where I could skate for ten to twenty miles. I ended up doing most of the distance skating on Madeline Island. Although I had never skated twenty-six miles, I had skated half that distance on the island, and I had read that if you can skate half a marathon, you could skate the whole thing. I decided to use that approach.

The day of the marathon I confess to being a little nervous since I had no idea what to expect. At 6 A.M. I boarded the bus that took us about twenty-five miles up Minnesota's scenic North Shore from Duluth to the starting area in Two Harbors. I nibbled a granola bar and sipped some water. I'm never a big water drinker, but I quickly noticed that nearly everyone else was consuming a lot of it. We arrived at Two Harbors, where I put on my skates and tossed shoes and jacket into a bag that would be returned to the finish area in Duluth. There were three classes of entrants: the pros, the advanced class, and the so-called citizen class (which would be renamed the recreational class in 1998). I learned that the pros skated in teams, are deadly serious about the competition, and generally finish in sixty to seventy minutes. That translated to a speed of twenty-five to twenty-eight miles per hour. The second wave is a bit slower. The citizen entrants seemed less concerned with time than with simply finishing. That was certainly my attitude.

It was a beautiful early-fall morning, and as I looked around, I realized I was one of nearly three thousand participants. After the first two classes started, our wave began to edge forward—slowly at first, then more quickly—because it took a while just to reach the starting line. I was beginning to feel exhilarated. Loudspeakers were blasting the *Rocky* theme as we crossed the start, which is on smooth blacktop that quickly slopes down a long, gentle incline so the skaters begin to move fast right at the start. I was part of a sea of humanity —men, women, kids, old, young, middle aged; all shapes and sizes, every imaginable skating outfit—everyone enjoying the high energy of the moment and keeping an eagle eye on other skaters, lest they have a collision early in the race.

I maintained a moderate pace for most of the race, taking a few sips of water at the aid stations and occasionally in between. For the first sixteen miles or so I was doing fine. At about the twenty-mile mark there was an uphill—not especially steep, but long—and by now I was tired and my skates felt like lead as I approached the top of the hill. That was followed by a downhill and a long stretch on Interstate 35, which, I discovered, is grooved pavement that sends vibrations up your legs and eventually makes your legs—mine, at least—feel like Jello. I barely made it up the exit ramp off the interstate and heard the volunteers tell us we had a quarter mile to go. I almost lost it on the final downhill, but pulled out of a near-stumble, did my best to sprint the final two hundred yards—and finished. I felt okay—tired, but a little dizzy, and I had trouble focusing my eyes. It was midmorning, and I knew I had to recover quickly and start back to Bayfield, because guests would be arriving by midafternoon. I sat down and rested, drank some water, ate oranges and yogurt, picked up my gear, and went to the car to start the hour-and-forty-five-minute drive home. But the parking lot and surrounding buildings were spinning. I started the engine, then said to myself, "This is crazy," turned it off and headed for the medical tent. They took my blood pressure and asked if I'd hydrated during the race. I learned that a few mouthfuls during the race doesn't qualify as proper hydration in a marathon. My blood pressure had plummeted, and as I lay on the medical cot for an hour with the IV in my arm, I realized I had learned a valuable lesson about water intake.

Since then I've returned to the Northshore Marathon twice, and both times made sure to get plenty of water, starting the day before the race. In 1998 we had a tailwind that made the times about fifteen minutes faster than the previous year. The first twenty pro racers all finished in sixty-five minutes or less. In 1999 I had what struck me as a funny, strange experience. I thought I had time to make one final Porta Potty stop, which isn't simple with skates on. While I was inside— seated—the national anthem began to play. Of course, we've all been taught to stand at attention when it's played. So I asked myself, Do I stand up? And will anyone know if I don't?

The 1999 race was different and important in another way. I had made a new friend, Katherine, who joined me in Duluth as my one-person cheering section and was waiting at the finish—an added incentive to complete the race.

In skating three marathons, I've learned the importance of taking care of myself if I want to continue competing. And I plan to continue: The date for 2000 is circled on my calendar. I've found that exercise helps me prioritize my life. As our lives become more complex—family, careers, friendships, personal activities—we become bogged down with multiple, and often competing, demands. Somewhere we must learn to budget time for ourselves and decide how to spend that time. For me, exercise needs to be part of that precious time. It might be biking, walking, or skating. But from spring to fall, I try hard to include skating as often as I can. It helps me maintain a sense of clarity in my life, and it helps me to get outside—especially when I get caught in the dizzying details of running the B&B. From mid-June to mid-September, I have a full house most days—eight guests. That means I'm up early to prepare breakfast, clean the house, do laundry, shop, chat with guests, tackle the ever-present bookwork—all the tasks that were to be shared, and now are done alone. Sometimes I'll be folding laundry at 2 P.M. and realize I haven't been outside yet, and I have guests arriving and shopping that must be done. So if I can, I'll put things on hold for an hour and try to get out for a skate or bike ride or just a walk.

I recommend inline skating for people of any age. It's a great activity if you approach it wisely. Get the right equipment and try it out before buying. Take a few lessons. Be sure to wear protective padding: helmet, wrist pads, knee pads, elbow pads. Learn to be a sensible skater, and it's a sport you can enjoy for many years. It can be fun on your own or as part of a group—whatever suits your style. And once you've developed confidence in your skills and your physical condition—well, you might consider trying a ten-miler, or a half marathon, or perhaps, someday, a marathon.

THE TWILIGHT YEARS

MANFRED D'ELIA

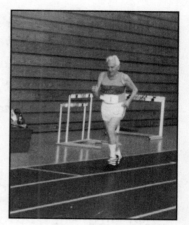

Date of birth 6-19-08

Residence: Ridgewood, New Jersey

"We do not count a man's years until there is nothing left to count." —Emerson

The great philosopher Satchel Paige once asked: "How old would you be if you didn't know how old you are?" This is a fitting question for Fred, who at ninety-one years old, lies about his age because he doesn't feel or look ninety-one. He wants to be eighty-two. Fred became a serious runner at age sixty-three and still runs competitively, but something has changed. Fred is in the early stages of Alzheimer's disease. It doesn't stop him from the physical activity he loves so much—his walks, daily track workouts with his wife, and the competitions. But he won't remember them. At times he is unable to recall a conversation he had an hour ago or sometimes even his wife of thirty years. But he still brings home medals and ribbons from the Senior Olympics. When I arrived for the interview, the sounds of Chopin's Nocturnes drifted through the room, creating a tranquil surrounding. Fred is a gifted pianist, one who feels the music in his heart before his fingers feel the ivory. Hundreds of credits to his musical career hang on the walls of his home. Other distinguished awards are also displayed for his accomplishments in track and mountain climbing. At age sixty-six, he ascended the Matterhorn. He has also climbed Mount Rainier, Mont Blanc, and in his seventies ascended Mount Damavand (over 18,000 feet) in Iran. Fred has a kind and humorous nature and the mannerisms of a gentleman. He truly is a man for all seasons.

I was born in 1908 in Paterson, New Jersey, which at the time was a mill town. That would make me 82 years old."

"No Fred, you are ninety-one. Stop telling Gail you're eighty-two."

"But Toshi, I don't feel ninety-one. I can still beat the pants off the old guys at the track. Show Gail my favorite medal, the one I got in high school. I am very proud of this. I won it in 1922 when I was fourteen for the hundred-yard dash at the Paterson High School Municipal Tournament. I didn't even know I could run then, but I guess I was fast."

"Tell Gail some things you remember about growing up."

"I am the second of four brothers. I think we are all still alive. Are we Toshi?"

"No, Fred. Only you and a younger brother are still alive."

"Well, I was a Boy Scout. I remember we held our meetings at the Protestant church, which I thought was kind of odd, being Catholic, but nobody cared, we were just a group of boys who liked doing things for the community—and hiking. That was a big part of our activities. We would go up into the Ramapo Mountains and hike all weekend. That's where I developed a love for the outdoors, especially the mountains. No one bothers you in the mountains. I always felt footloose and free out there. Later on, when I was living in Europe I would always have my hiking shoes thrown over my shoulders and would tag along with the local townsfolk when they headed up into the hiking trails."

"Fred, you're skipping over too much. Tell Gail about your parents."

"Well, they came over from Italy by way of Argentina to Paterson. My father was an ironworker and had a successful business in Suffern. We used to take the trolley up from Paterson. The place is still there today, but none of my brothers wanted that. My oldest brother became a doctor, I went into music, and another received an appointment to West Point. My brother George, five years younger than me, worked in the Brooklyn Naval Yard. He was a gentle, religious man who took care of Poppa until he died at ninety-four. George passed away in 1983.

"After high school I got a job at a bank in New York, but then the depression hit and just about everyone was let go. I had been taking piano lessons and sometimes would supplement my wages by playing at lunchtime. The bank president heard me play and suggested that I concentrate on my music instead of banking. He felt that I had a talent that shouldn't be wasted. Because of his encouragement, I went to Italy to study piano. It was the best piece of advice I ever took. Not only was I doing what I loved, but also it gave me the opportunity to see other parts of Europe. On weekends I would travel to the Alps, Bulgaria, anywhere that I could climb. Unfortunately, my travels in Europe were cut short due to Mussolini's army. As a second-generation Italian, I was eligible for the draft. Mussolini's soldiers were desperate for bodies for his escalating war effort and I was targeted. My landlord warned me the soldiers were on their way and I ran. I just picked up and left.

"Back in the States I got a job as musical director of a church and slowly began to build a roster of students and soon was able to open my own music school. I was very fortunate that I could select from the most dedicated and gifted of students. Many of them have gone on to distinguish themselves in their field. I think right about then I married Toshi, is that right?"

"Yes, we got married in 1962."

"Wow, that long ago? You mean I've put up with you all those years? I must deserve a medal for that."

"You have it wrong, Fred. I'm the one who deserves the medal."

"After we married, I would take Toshi on my hikes. It was wonderful to have her as a companion."

"What do you mean, companion? I was your donkey. You only brought me along to carry all the gear. But I didn't mind. You were in better shape than I was so I needed to work at getting stronger. I carried the gear as a way of strength training. That's also when I started running so I could increase my endurance. Our daughter was running track at the high school and decided to teach me how to run. One day when we returned from a workout at the track, Fred showed us his 1922 medal. My daughter was so impressed that she talked him into joining us at the track. It became our family project. Erica, our coach, decided we were ready for some competition and entered us in the World Masters Track and Field Championships in Toronto. This was back in 1975. I was forty-five and Fred was sixty-seven. We had a wonderful time, and Fred came home with a silver medal in the hundred-meter and a bronze medal in the two hundred."

"I was in good shape. I remember an old Scotsman at the

event who was ninety-four years old. We were all amazed that he could even stand up, let alone run. I said to Toshi, 'Look at that old man out there running around the track.' Now I *am* that old man.

"We competed in this event every two years until ten years ago. But I still compete in the eastern regionals. I tend to win, because there is no one else alive in my division. Sometimes I have to run with the younger guys in the eighty-to-eighty-five division because I have no one to compete against. And I usually beat them! Toshi coaches me now, and she's tough."

"You must be joking, Fred. I'm more your nursemaid now than coach. We go to the track every other day and work out. If the weather is good, we'll go outdoors to the high school, but if it's inclement or winter, we go to an indoor track. I have my own workout routine, which is too hard for Fred so he'll just walk a lap or two to warm up. Then I hand him his track shoes, he slips then on, I lace him up, and he is ready. I'm not sure he really needs these racing flats, but it makes him feel special, puts him in the mood to run. He'll do some light speed work, jog a little, then walk again. If I'm still working out and need more time, Fred never gets bored. He keeps busy by cleaning up the track area. He'll walk around picking up trash. He says it is his civic responsibility, but then he puts all the trash in my pockets to carry home!"

"I never worry about stretching. At my age I don't worry about those things anymore. I do whatever I want. I was born with good genes and that's what it boils down to. No matter how much I train or stretch or work out, if it's not in the genes, it's not there."

"Just this past March, I entered Fred in the Eastern Regionals Indoor Track and Field Meet in New York. There was no one else competing in his age group so he ran with the eighty-year-olds, which was just as well because Fred was up to his tricks again telling everyone he was eighty-two. I was actually questioned by the officials for putting his age down as ninety-one. He doesn't look it or act it, so they were suspicious of me. The track had a rather high incline at the outermost lane, where they put Fred, and I thought he was going to tip over. He did the fifty-meter dash in 18 seconds and the two-hundred-meter dash in 1:01. He always receives the loudest applause, especially when they learn he is ninety-one."

"I'm not ninety-one, I'm eighty-two. I refuse to be ninety-one. It's too old. I'm just starting to live. I still have all my teeth, which is surely a sign of good health, and I eat whatever the boss puts in front of me. I am very easy to get along with and I don't worry about things. Heck, there's always someone who is more than willing to worry for me about things, so why should I bother? I hated to give up hiking and climbing but I had to admit that my footing was getting risky. I miss it. I loved being out in the woods, watching the trees, the streams, the rocks. It beats looking at cars and traffic all day. It was a pure enjoyment, a marvelous way to spend time. But it was time to quit and now I feel lucky just to get out for a walk. That's all it really takes anyway. Walking is a great exercise.

"I know there are people who seem to stop enjoying life when they reach a certain age. When you reach your fifties or sixties, exercise does become more of an effort. Your body is not twenty anymore. It takes discipline. But more than that, it takes desire. You have to want it. The desire has to be there or nothing will get you out the door. I can still get around; I have no worries, no negative thoughts. But then again, I'm not that old yet. My father lived to ninety-four. I look young, act young, and I'm with younger people all the time. Toshi will sometimes take me to her running club meetings and I love seeing everyone. They say, 'Hey Fred, you look terrific,' and it makes my day."

"What Fred didn't tell you is that he started that running club in 1975 as a way for people to run and train together, to share a common interest. We started the club with 19 members and today have over 250. He also didn't tell you that he still teaches piano. He has one student who still insists on seeing Fred. It truly is amazing. His mind doesn't function from hour to hour, yet he can sit at the piano and know every key, every exercise, and every note. The musical section of his brain is solidly intact. He always said to me when we were first married and struggling along, 'The music in my blood is better than any money in the bank.' His attitude is what keeps me sane now that I am caring for him all the time. There are so many positive things about him, but his attitude is everything. I know some other wives my age and in my situation whose husbands have turned bitter and nasty. It's a very sad thing to watch. Fred cares about his appearance and he tries to be receptive to my suggestions. If he balks, I tell him he'd look ten times more handsome if he did what I suggested, and that usually works. He enjoys being with others, even if he can't remember their names or recall the conversation. He doesn't want to be shut away and become a recluse. When that happens, you lose the desire to live."

"I take life one day at a time. I have a number of activities I still enjoy doing such as running, walking, and playing the piano. Young people today should take advantage of all the opportunities they have. I grew up during the depression, lived through two world wars and countless other wars. They weren't always the best of times, but we made them good. You take advantage of what you have and kids today have far more than I ever did. This country has so many opportunities. Whether it's hiking, climbing, running, or playing the piano, whatever it is will teach kids valuable lessons in discipline and effort for life. All you have to do is want it."

Postscript: Fred died peacefully in his sleep at home in March 2000. His memorial service was attended by many friends of all ages, a multigenerational gathering of people who knew and loved Fred. It was a moving service, a tribute to a great and gentle man who left behind a legacy of kindness and dedication to his family, friends, and passions.

A FREE SPIRIT WITH RUNNING SHOES

PIERRE DELFAUSSE

Date of birth: 1-10-17

Residence: Carmel-by-the-Sea, California

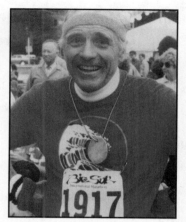

> **"Old boys have their playthings as well as young ones; the difference is only in the price." —Benjamin Franklin**

Pierre just may be the last of the free spirits. Maybe it was all the years he spent in the toy industry that keeps his outlook on life young and innocent. Growing up in the depression, he went on to be a very successful businessman. He retired at fifty-seven, gave away most of his money and all his earthly possessions, and moved to California. At eighty-five years old, he finds the simple life suits him just fine. His home is a rented garage, which he shared with a big golden retriever. When he's not jogging on the beach at Carmel or working at his job as a gardener and caretaker at a Pebble Beach estate, he can be found running or volunteering at the Big Sur International Marathon, which he has run eight times.

Sport was always a big factor in our house as my father was a coach of the New York Nationals basketball team back in 1908. They were considered the world champions during his tenure. My mother actually had the harder job, as she had to raise four boys. We lived on Long Island and managed to survive the flu epidemic of 1917, which wiped out almost the entire community. I have to admit I was a jock in high school, captain of the soccer team, and ended up with more varsity letters than anyone in the history of the school. And of course we all played basketball. Couldn't avoid that. But my real love was skiing. There was a small ski area in the Poconos called the Inn at Buckhill Falls, which had a rope tow. It was quite primitive compared to today's ski resorts, but a mountain is a mountain. It just took longer to get to the top. Stowe, Vermont was also open to skiers, but again with only a rope tow.

Getting out of high school in 1935, there were no jobs due to the depression, so it was back to school for postgraduate work, which really meant one more year of playing soccer and basketball. Everybody had odd jobs during that time and I was no different, making fifteen dollars a week dishing out soft ice cream at a frozen custard stand. My dad had left the basketball association in 1910 and was working in the toy business as a factory representative but that company went bankrupt, as did most depression-era businesses, so my father struck out on his own in 1930.

The army came calling in 1943, but my wife had just delivered our first child so they gave me a month off before being shipped out. On the draft notice I listed skiing as my hobby and was assigned to the Tenth Mountain Division Ski Troops. We were shipped off to Camp Hale in Colorado, ten thousand feet above sea level, a beautiful spot that just happen to be the back side of Vail. After completing the training, the next stop was Texas for jungle training. Our destination was supposed to be the Burma Road in Asia, but instead we were sent to the Apennine Mountains in Italy. We arrived in January, started combat one month later, and finished the mission by April. It was quite an incredible experience. The only way in or out of the area was to climb sheer cliffs. No one ever thought it was possible to do what we did. It took its toll on us though, as there were many casualties, me included, although mine was more of a mishap than a casualty. We were in Villa Franca and I was riding with our commander in his jeep ahead of the platoon. The truck behind our jeep didn't take notice that we had stopped or that I was getting out of the jeep, so I found myself slammed up against a wall and just about crushed by the truck. The accident separated my shoulder and caused serious contusions of the back. I had to be flown home to the army hospital in Colorado and received a medical discharge. The injury slowed me down for a few years but eventually healed. During the war it wasn't uncommon to come under attack from your own side by accident. I remember pulling a horse-drawn cart filled with ammunition to the front line when suddenly our own flyboys swooped down from the air and opened up with machine gun fire at us as we jumped for cover. From the air we must have looked like Germans.

Back home in 1945 I took over the toy business from my father, whose health was failing;he died shortly after. I built the business up from scratch, eventually employing fifteen agents. I traveled all over the United States, Europe, Japan, anywhere there was business. There was no time for sports or exercise of any kind. The toy industry was taking off in leaps and bounds in 1961 with the advent of major products like the hula hoop, followed by Hasbro's GI Joe and the Duncan Yo-Yo. It was an exciting time but business kept me on the road. New toys were being introduced all over the place. The first time I saw kids in California playing with a hula hoop, I ran to the phone to call New York and tried to describe what I was seeing and they thought I was crazy. It was already a hot craze on the West Coast, but New York had no idea what was about to hit them. The Duncan yo-yo received an even bigger introduction in the toy business. Demonstrations and promotional ideas were my forte and I was always looking for ways to promote items. One particular year, 1965, I was introducing a hockey game right before Thanksgiving at Macy's and had to hire and train unemployed actors for demonstrations and sales. Remember, this was pre–Toys "R" Us, and the major department stores were one of the few places to buy toys. It used to be a big event to unveil the toy department right after Thanksgiving. We used the out-of-work actors because we could get away with paying them fifteen dollars a day—plus they were always available. I ended up hiring one young, unemployed actor who always seemed to have a cold, wheezed, and was very unprepossessing. But he was a warm body and I needed a demonstrator. Even had to buy him a Montreal Canadiens hockey jersey before he went on the job. Whenever I went to check on him at Macy's he was never there. He was either on a break or had just left. The other demonstrators covered for him, but eventually I got fed up, and two weeks later I fired Dustin Hoffman. Years later we met at a party and he introduced me to others as his first boss.

I was having a lot of fun, but the downside was no time for physical activity. *Sedentary* best describes my level of sports participation during this phase of my life. Turning fifty seemed like the pinnacle of my life, and to celebrate the milestone I decided to take a trip to New Zealand and Australia. I truly thought I was getting old and would die soon. My dad died at sixtry-two, so there was no reason not to think I'd follow in his footsteps. If I didn't go then, I'd never get there. Nowadays the perception of aging has greatly changed for the better. Fifty is young compared to the way we looked at it. Especially for athletes who had no choice but to give up and let the younger ones take over. There were no age divisions back then. When you got too old to compete, you quit. Today, most senior athletes can't wait to move up to the next age division—to turn fifty and compete in an age bracket where they are the youngest. There's always something to look forward to. If I had the chance to turn fifty all over again, I'd probably celebrate it by running a marathon or playing in a tennis tournament.

Eventually the constant work and travel took their toll on me and in 1973 I quit. Gave it up. Retired at fifty-seven and never looked back. I was tired of New York, tired of the toy business, and tired of working twelve-hour days. I was making a six-figure salary but gave it all away—that and the house—when I got a divorce and moved to California with nothing but my freedom, a dropout. Arriving in Carmel free of possessions, I found an apartment in a garage, got a job as a gardener and couldn't have been happier.

Getting back in shape was my first priority, so I started jogging. I won't even call it running; just jogs along the beach, maybe two miles. Carmel is a runners' paradise, and the beaches were the perfect spot to start. Life was perfect for a while. It was nice to sleep late, walk the beaches, sip a good cup of coffee while reading the *Times*. But too much of that can become boring! Checking out the local classified ads, I took a job as a caretaker for a family that live on a large estate in Pebble Beach. It was the perfect job and as a benefit, I was outdoors. In the meantime my jogging was turning into a decent run and when I turned sixty-six I graduated into a runner. What was the difference? My first race. Another runner I met on the beach suggested we enter a local 10K, and even though I didn't know what that was, it sounded like fun. That first race was all it took; I was hooked. To date I've run 250 races. After enough 5Ks and 10Ks, I had to tackle a marathon and put in my application for the Big Sur International Marathon, not too far from my home. It was 1986 and I was sixty-nine years old. Big Sur is one of the most beautiful courses on the marathon circuit, but hilly with high winds at the crest. It brought back my ski trooper days, only this time I wasn't using skis to scale a mountain, I was running it. Some of the comparisons to mountain climbing are the same, literally and figuratively. We climb mountains because they are there and runners run marathons because they are there. In fact, I had such a good time at Big Sur, I went back the following year and cut my time to 4:43, winning the seventy and over men's division. If you make something fun, anything, it won't be a chore, won't become boring. For example, when I enter a race I always request my birth-date, 1917, as my bib number. It's just a little thing, but it makes it more fun. To date, I've run the Big Sur International Marathon eight times and when I'm not running, I volunteer.

At eighty-two years old, I still enjoy all the pleasures of a race whether competing or volunteering. It's hard to get competition at my age. When I was running for time, I was always trying to figure out who was passing me and what age division they might be in. Were they in my age category? Were they contenders? Did I have to run faster to beat them? Most of the time I'd give up, thinking someone in my division had passed me, but when I got to the finish I'd find out they were ten years younger! Go figure. I'm still winning.

There's nothing like running for cleansing the mind or problem solving. It doesn't matter how fast or slow I run. That's not why I do it. It keeps me fit and it keeps me happy. Two months ago I underwent arthroscopic knee surgery to replace worn and torn cartilage but I didn't let it get me down. In fact, four weeks later I entered a 5K race using my crutches and won my age group. Age is but a quality of mind. If you leave your dreams behind, what do you have? All my life I've done what I wanted to do. The toy business kept me young and I guess I never grew up. The widow I care for in the estate at Pebble Beach is ninety. When I'm not caring for her, I volunteer at our local community hospital, mostly pushing people around in wheelchairs. When I'm not at the hospital or managing the estate, I play with my dogs. My home is half of a garage, a space about twenty-two feet by twelve feet. It's perfect. I share it with my big golden retriever. No matter where I'm sitting, I can reach out and pet her. There used to be three big goldens, but two passed away recently. Everything I need is within my reach, everything I want is at my fingertips. People get too caught up with possessions and it can ruin their outlook on what is important in life. There's a passage in the New Testament, Matthew 6:9, that goes something like, "Lay you not treasures on earth where moth and rust doth corrupt and where thieves break in and steal." I have no worries. I can't remember a morning that I didn't wake up happy. And after a relaxing weekend, I can't wait for Mondays because it means I get to go back to work!

More people are living to a hundred than ever before. The *Today* show used to announce people's birthday when they reached ninety, but now they've had to move it up to a hundred because there are so many ninety-year-olds out there. That tells you something. There are more outlets for people my age to participate in sports, like the Fifty-Plus club. There's no reason why people of any age shouldn't be in shape. But obesity is on the rise in some age groups in America and I can't understand that. I blame some of it on corporate America, too many people working too hard and not getting any exercise. At the hospital where I volunteer, we've had to buy extra-wide wheelchairs to accommodate some of the obese patients. That's a real concern for our country. We're overfed. When I turned sixty-two, I became a vegetarian. I don't smoke and never indulged in alcohol. Coca-Cola is my big downfall. The real difference in how people age is vitality, and that comes with exercise and a positive frame of mind. That doesn't mean everyone has to become an elite athlete, so to speak. Remember Jack LaLanne? He taught people how to exercise using a chair.

Keeping busy and feeling there is a purpose to your life is the key to successful aging. I don't think I'll ever get old.

COUCH POTATO AT 50, JOCK AT 63

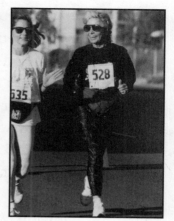

ROSEMARY ENNIS, Ph.D.

Date of birth: 7-2-31

Residence: La Jolla, California

> **"You don't get to choose how you are going to die.
> Or when. You can only decide how you are going to live."**
> **—Joan Baez**

A self-described duffer, Rosemary was never an athlete. Back in school she was never chosen for a team at recess or in gym. But she made up for lost timewhen she became an athlete in her sixties. She ran her first marathon at sixty-eight and just returned from summiting Mount Kilimanjaro. Receiving her Ph.D. in nutrition at sixty-five, she has written a book about successful aging, a compendium of good health. According to Ennis, the first thing you must do is change your beliefs and attitudes regarding aging and get more positive on the subject. Exercise and nutrition have turned her life around, and she is living proof that they can do the same for you.

Sport was never a part of my growing up. When I was two we moved from New York to Chicago, where my grandparents and all my mom's brothers and sisters lived. It was during the Depression but my dad always worked and I don't remember being deprived very much, except for having holey socks. My parents enrolled me in a Polish Catholic school. Polish was never spoken by any of our relatives, and my mom wanted to show me off as being able to speak a second language. She was always in competition with her siblings and their kids, my cousins. Of course my grandparents were thrilled, and it really wasn't that hard at age five to pick up the language. I learned reading, writing, arithmetic and catechism in Polish. I remember being sick with earaches and sore throats a lot back then and missing about half of the school year but I still excelled in scholastics, but never sports. I earned a holy picture card for being at the top of my first-grade class.

When I was nine my dad came to California to work for the war effort. My two younger brothers, little sister, and I were thrilled. San Diego was a heavenly paradise in February compared to Chicago. Blue skies, green palm trees, orange trees, and yellow lemon trees all in full bloom in the middle of winter. We even went swimming at La Jolla cove and it seemed warmer than Lake Michigan in summer.

I couldn't wait to enroll in school. However, I was never athletic, never had any interest in sports. Nobody ever chose me for their team at recess or in gym. Sports were a real bugaboo for me. Could never run fast enough, hit the ball hard enough, was always the one left behind. It was humiliating, and I tried to get out of gym to avoid the embarrassment of not being chosen or finishing last. I volunteered for bathroom monitor duty and crossing-guard patrol just to avoid gym. As a side benefit I became a bookworm so that I had an excuse for not doing sports. Ironically enough, at the close of my senior year in high school I was the first female and nonathlete to win the school trophy, which was based on the highest number of points earned for sports, social accomplishments such as being president of a club or on the student council, and academic merit. Up until then, 1948, it always was awarded to the top male athlete because he usually accumulated the most points.

At San Diego State University, I signed up for archery, swimming, and square dancing as my required gym classes, still avoiding anything athletic. At nineteen I married a basketball and track star, Chuck Boucher, and quit school to take a job to support my husband while he finished college. The idea was that after he received his degree in education and got a job, I would continue my education in psychology. Ah, the best-laid plans. Along the way, we had four children. By the time the fourth child was born, the oldest was only three. I was also going to school at night to finish my degree. Then we divorced. But no matter what life had in store for me, I always continued my education. That took a very long time, but I finally received my bachelor's degree in psychology, and then continued on to a master's in physiological psychology and another in health science at age sixty. I earned my doctorate of philosophy in nutrition at sixty-five. Slow learner, but steady.

Marrying a second time, I fell for another athlete. Brice Ennis was a natural. When we bought a ski boat, I spent all summer trying to get up on two skis. At Brice's first attempt, he popped off the beach and was up and away on one ski. Hated that. When he took up running, his first race was a 26.2-mile marathon. His first bicycle race was a century (one hundred miles). Remember that I was still raising four babies, the eldest of whom was now six. I didn't have much time for sports, but I did try tennis. Always the perennial beginner, I gave it up because no one would play with me. Brice and I had a child, bringing the menagerie to five. I was also still working and going to school so there was not much time for anything, much less sports.

It's a funny thing about aging. When I reached my fifties I noticed that Brice was becoming more athletic and better looking. He was always extremely handsome, but now he was downright gorgeous. On the other hand, I was becoming quite frumpy, sort of square shaped and flabby. In the morning he'd spring out of bed for his morning run and I'd just lie there with the pillow over my head hiding deeper and deeper under the covers. I tried very hard not to do anything that would raise my heart count. But at fifty-three I couldn't stand my floppy self anymore and decided to do something about it. I looked about for a magic pill but none were available. Running seemed the most logical, as I didn't need a partner, a set time, or any special equipment. I just pulled on my dime store sneakers and ran for a hundred steps. I counted all the steps because I couldn't wait till it was over. That was enough for my first week of exercise. I hated it. I was exhausted. The second week I made it to a hundred and five steps three times a week. It took me a year to work up to a mile. Then I entered my first 5K race because I was motivated by the beer and orange slices served at the finish. Seemed like a good reason for drinking beer in the morning to me. That race was the most difficult thing I ever did in my life. More difficult than having babies. It's just not easy for me. I remembered my Catholic school Polish prayers and prayed for the angels to lift me up and carry me to the finish.

As I entered more races, I began to look and feel better, and I always came home with a medal or trophy regardless of how slowly I ran, back of the pack, because no women my age were running races in those days. The kids and Brice loved the new me and were very supportive. Now they just yawn and say, "Ho-hum, Mom won another race." But daughter number three, Val, did meet me at the end of my first marathon recently and there were no ho-hums, just lots of tears and feeling proud.

Winning the medals was thrilling and I'd forget how bad I felt during the race. All enthusiastic, I'd sign up for the next race. Then it would all come back and I'd be running and thinking, "Why am I here? Why am I doing this? My back hurts, my feet hurt, I can't breathe, I'm running as fast as I can but everyone is passing me—even the race walkers. The mile markers must be wrong." Then I'd get the medal and forget all the woes all over again. I kept at it because I knew it was good for me, but more importantly I could eat whatever I wanted. I never had to diet again. Hooray! Worth the price of admission. To this day, though, I still hate exercising.

Cycling. Another challenge and a half. My first distance bike race was 125 miles. I trained zero miles. It's actually like a big weekend party in Ensenada, Mexico, so once again I was motivated. Partying is one of the things I do best. The course begins in Mexicali, Mexico, with about ten thousand participants. I just get on the bike and go. Brice told me, "You're amazing," especially when some of the well-trained men drop out half way. I try to forget how long it takes to ride 125 miles and sing Christmas carols in Polish. Since I am on a tandem with Brice, he hurries to the finish to avoid my singing, which is really bad.

Next, Brice entered the Huntsman World Senior Games in St. George, Utah. I was a tagalong because I love trips, anytime, anywhere. We went for two days and two nights but stayed for a week, bought a house, and I moved there half time. I looked up at smog-free blue skies, watched people leave their cars with the windows open and the doors unlocked, talked with little kids who greeted me first, and finally turned to Brice and said, "I don't know what you're doing, but I'm staying here." Since Brice's job was mainly traveling, we had the flexibility to call anyplace home.

Brice had signed up for the biking time trials, which were held in the frontier town of Enterprise, Utah. If I had to do it all over again, I'd raise my kids in Enterprise. I came along just to watch but got immediately caught up with the frenzy and enthusiasm of the senior cyclists. This is a very dangerous sport, but these old guys and gals couldn't care less. Dauntless! They were truly amazing. Of all the two thousand competitors in St. George, the cyclists seemed to be in the best condition. Ernie Marinoni was ninety-one then; he's ninety-six now and still racing. The next year I became cycling director. I knew nothing about cycling but I am an excellent administrator and organizer. I did this for five years before resigning and becoming a competitor in the 5K and 10K races and the triathlon. Last year I was the running member of a three-person team, but the previous two years I'd done the swimming, cycling and running on my own— slowly of course, but I was old enough to win. The triathlon consists of a 5K run, a 500-meter swim and a 20K bike course. I beat eighty-eight-year-old Ralph from New York, and that was good enough for me.

I can analyze the reasons I began exercising at fifty-three and continue to stay in shape three different ways. First, I like to eat and gain weight easily. Once I started running I never had to diet—and believe me, I dieted my whole life. You name the diet and I was on it. I've never been a junk eater, always been health conscious, but I'm not real strict. I do stay away from sugar; it has such an adverse affect on sleeping, thinking, the muscles and joints. My Ph.D. is in nutrition and I've come a long way in my dietary recommendations. I work mostly with older athletes, and cutting out sugar makes them go faster with fewer injuries. I haven't had a cold or a bout with the flu in over twenty-five years. I was a true believer and promoter of anti-oxidants long before they became popular. Used to embarrass my kids no end. I take just about everything there is . . . handfuls every morning . . . and some just in case. My favorites are ester C and calcium—which by the way is best taken at night before bedtime, because calcium absorption is difficult.

Second, at my age I need to increase my muscle mass and avoid the pitfalls of osteoporosis. And who wants flab? Yuck. Unattractive. I've been able to maintain a body-fat ratio of 17 percent. A woman of any age is lucky to have a body-fat ratio of 22 percent. Exercise is the key here and since I hate exercise, I run a little, walk a lot, and lift weights a little bit, do yoga stretches now and then.

Third, exercise is mental vacation. Everyone has stress and problems and exercise offers a time to work things through and alleviate the stress. Got a problem? Get out there and walk or run or bike. You'll feel much better. Research documents the results. Not only is running or walking satisfying and healthy, researchers have shown that the immune system is enhanced. The pituitary glands secrete the hormones that not only give runners a natural high but also enhance the white blood cell count, which improves the immune system.

So now there is a scientific explanation for what most of us know instinctively.

Speaking of a runner's high, as I mentioned earlier, I ran my first marathon this past year at age sixty-eight. It didn't seem like that great an accomplishment because I am such a duffer. It was just one more thing like raising five kids five years apart, always working toward a degree, and then another and another, and working full time and having fifteen grandchildren (that was the easiest part of my life). I guess these goals keep me off the streets (except when I am running) and out of the pool halls. Oh, and it rained on my first marathon, first rain San Diego had had in a year. But it was worse on the people waiting for me at the finish. I ran between the drops; they stood there and got soaked. Running a marathon, like any other challenge in life, is part attitude, part training. I remember thinking back to having a hard time running a 10K; the thought of a marathon seemed insurmountable. If you set a goal, whether or not you think you can achieve it, you *can* attain it. Setting it is the key. The rest just follows. Make your brain work with your body. They are partners, and without that relationship the task is going to be tougher. I am as lazy as I can be and don't ever look forward to my next run or next bike race. I do it because I know it is good for me. The key is making it simple and pain-free. I am not a proponent of the "no pain, no gain" philosophy. Just the opposite. My mantra is "no pain, no pain." If it hurts, don't do it, slow down. Train your body to endure and accept more pressure, more distance, not more pain.

One of my greatest achievements in the health field was being one in five selected from 500 U.S. applicants to address the First International Symposium on Healthy Lifestyles, sponsored by the United Nations and held in St. Petersburg, Russia. I also teach seminars on "Looking Good, Feeling Great." It's important to spread that message and help motivate others. I've written a book called *Just Say Whoa to Aging*, which is based on the mind, attitudes, nutrition, and exercise guidelines as the best way to fight the so-called "diseases" of aging. My credentials are impressive: a couch potato at fifty, semi-superjock at sixty. The reason to do any of this stuff is not to live longer but to have a zest for life until I die. I've put twenty years of research into pursuing the idea that a healthy mind, spirit, and body can result in a more abundant and rewarding life. Next time you run a race, pick one with the best goodie bag or best T-shirt, not the one where you'll kill yourself trying for a P.R. At my age, if I can't put a smile on my face when crossing the finish line, then I'm not having any fun and something is wrong.

These are important messages as our population gets older. Our beliefs and emotions influence our brain's chemistry and therefore our state of health. Smiling and laughing should be classified as a mandatory exercise. It is something we should do to each other and ourselves every day. It takes no special equipment. Just set a goal to feel the best you can, look the best you can, and *be* the best you can, every day without pain. It's up to you. Just know that it is doable. My next challenge is climbing Mount Kilimanjaro. As far as I know, if I succeed in my goal I will be the oldest woman to summit—and of course, *I will summit!*

LITTLE ABNER

JOE GOLD

Date of birth: 3-10-22

Residence: Santa Monica,
California

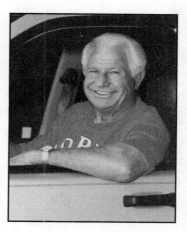

**"Do you know what the greatest test of life is?
Ask yourself if you still get excited about what you do
when you get up in the morning." —David Halberstam**

You can't get any busier than Joe Gold. It took me months to nail down a time this seventy-eight-year-old could spend with me on the phone. If he wasn't at a meeting for his chain of World Gyms, he was at a construction site going over the plans for new office space. One of the original Muscle Beach bodybuilders, Joe has dedicated his life to his profession. In one sense he has never left the beach: His office is just a few miles down the road from the famed Muscle Beach in Santa Monica, California. He fought in the wars, was a Hollywood stuntman, and was an original member of the Mae West Traveling Nightclub Show. Joe is one guy who has truly seen the world and has no regrets. He recently broke his arm in a fall and considers it nothing but a nuisance. It will mend. He is still best friends with his high school buddies, the same ones who gave him that nickname!

My nickname as a kid was 'Little Fat Boy.' At age twelve, I was already overweight and wanted to change. Started with changing my diet and using weights and by seventeen had a pretty good body and a new nickname, Little Abner. I made my own weights, as you couldn't buy a lot of weight equipment back then. The body is an amazing machine; if you give it the go-ahead, it will work with you. All you have to do is put in the time and eat a proper diet.

My best buddies, Harold Zinkin, Bob Tucker, and I started working out at the pier on the beach near Long Beach and in Santa Monica. Our goal was to get good enough to work our way up to the famed Muscle Beach. The guys who worked out there were a bit ahead of us, and we wanted to tone our acts before joining that crowd. Harold was the best athlete of the three of us and he was already primed. I wasn't a natural and therefore had to work harder, but I never got discouraged. I much preferred volleyball to making human pyramids but I had broad shoulders and loved the beach so it all came together. Soon we were all Muscle Beach regulars. It was 1939 and the beach was in full bloom. Everyone from Jack LaLanne to Vic and Armand Tanny worked out at the beach. Although the stunts and bodybuilding exhibitions were incredible, the most important thing at Muscle Beach was the friendships we made. I kept working out all through high school. In fact, I established my first gym in an old garage while still in junior high, The Dugout Athletic Club. It got its name because it was carved into the side of a hill on our property.

When the war broke out, Harold and I planned to enlist together but his plans got changed and he was sent to physical instruction and rehabilitation school to become a physical therapist. I enlisted in the Coast Guard in 1942, spending three years, five months, and twenty-nine days on tour, two years of which were spent in the fighting zone out in the South Pacific. After the South Pacific I served in the Aleutian Islands for a few months. I was very lucky to also be stationed on a military watch on the Santa Monica Pier. It was a great time. The point of mentioning this is that there were some good times during the war; it wasn't all bad. However, one of the bad times was during a bombing raid while in the South Pacific. I took a fall that caused spinal injuries. Returning to the States I was sent to a rehabilitation hospital and Harold Zinkin was my therapist. Small world. The residual effects of the spinal cord injury have made it necessary for me to use a wheelchair since 1980. But that doesn't stop me. I don't let anything stop me. I have no complaints. I've seen the world. And in between wars and the merchant marines, there was always the beach to come back to. When we weren't pulled away by wars or other disasters, at least six months of every year was spent at the beach. We'd all be there together. Everything centered around the beach when we were young. In some ways I've never left the beach. Still live right by it. I just can't take as much sun as I did as a kid.

Right after the war I swore I'd collect my 52-20, which was veteran's pay of twenty dollars a week for fifty-two weeks. But it didn't quite cover all my costs, so I decided to try the merchant marines, where I served from 1948 to 1978. A lot of the Muscle Beach regulars returning from the war signed on in Hollywood as stunt doubles. Show business was a natural for us, as we had already performed our bodybuilding stunts in front of thousands at the beach. I was no exception and became a stunt double. In 1954 we got word that Mae West was putting together a nightclub act and was looking for nine bodybuilders. She was sixty-two at the time and wanted to surround herself with young, handsome bodybuilders. I liked her and the $250 a week I would be earning, so I signed on. After ten months of a one-year commitment, I was caught kissing one of the camera girls, which did not please Mae West. She considered us her boys and if we wanted to do anything, it had to be with her. Shortly after the kissing incident I was fired, but then rehired in 1956. Quit again and was rehired in 1959. But finally I quit for good and returned to the beach. It was a lot of fun, an exciting time in my life. I got to see the nightclub limelight from the backstage side. Mae was a great woman. We got along despite all the firing and rehiring.

I opened my first official gym in New Orleans in 1952 with my partner, Charles Krauser—aka Paul Novak—who was Mae West's last lover. He stayed with her until she died in 1980. I have lots of memorabilia of the Mae West days that he willed to me upon his death this past year. Chuck and I sailed in the merchant marines together, went to the Korean War together, and even did a stint as professional wrestlers. We both needed to get away for a while, so we drove to Miami Beach. We lay on the beach for a few months and decided we needed something new to do. That turned out to be our first gym, called Ajax. We chose New Orleans because Vic and Armand Tanny already had California sewed up with their chain of Vic Tanny's Gyms.

Back in Santa Monica in 1959, Muscle Beach was essentially destroyed. That hurt. I organized the regulars and together we launched a Muscle Beach Weightlifting Gym, a nonprofit corporation. It worked for a while but we had to keep changing locations. So I decided to go it alone and opened Gold's Gym in 1964 at 106 Pacific Avenue in Venice. I built the structure and all of the equipment myself. It was a no mercy kind of gym for people who were serious about their body-building. I sold the gym in 1970, and the new owners kept the name and developed it into an international chain. Meanwhile, I returned to the merchant marines for another tour of duty.

A few years later I began World Gym, which I still own and operate out of the main location in Venice. I've been around this business a long time and have dedicated my life to it. Starting out doing it for myself to lose weight and develop muscle, it became a routine for life. Now I am passing on that knowledge to others. In recent years I've seen a huge increase in the number of older people joining gyms. It's a chance for them to turn back the clock on aging through exercise. It's a very important part of the aging process and there is scientific proof to back up the fact that older people who exercise look and feel younger than their age implies.

The average age of my gym clientele is fifty. The most sought-after pieces of equipment at the gyms are the cardio-vascular ones such as the treadmill and stationary bikes. Positive and welcome industry changes have been made to accommodate the older crowd, but still more can and should be done. I've been after the manufacturers of hand weights to make their equipment with more increments so you don't have to go from a five-pound dumbbell up to a ten. People need to increase their weights slowly, especially women and seniors. You can't just jump into an exercise program and expect immediate results. By starting out slowly and pro-gressing at a steady rate, you should avoid injuries. And everyone needs to be responsible, both the gym employees and the client.

I'm pushing eighty and if I can use myself as an example, I

look and feel much younger than my age. Even with my physical hardships of the spinal cord and being in a wheelchair, I am a very strong person. Just recently I broke my arm but it hasn't stopped me. I have plenty of vitality. I can't say enough about the positive role exercise plays throughout life. It doesn't matter when you start, as long as you do it.

WORKING OUT IN TOP HAT AND TAILS

RALPH GUILD

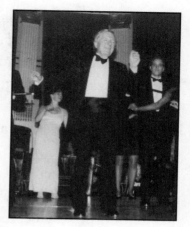

Date of birth: 9-11-28

Residence: Palm Beach, Florida

"The essence of age is intellect." —Emerson

As an only child of divorced parents growing up in the depression era, Ralph found comfort in books, musicals, and radio shows. Sports never held an interest for him, but a good Fred Astaire movie or listening to a radio comedy could make his day. Blessed with a strong determination and sharp mind, he worked his way up from cutting lawns to radio DJ, radio sales, and finally running his own international corporation. And instead of picking up golf or tennis in middle age, he started tap dance lessons on his fiftieth birthday and has been tapping ever since. At seventy-one, he finds that a daily workout combining tap, jazz, ballroom, and a good dose of stretching keeps him mentally and physically fit as a fiddle. With no plans for retirement, he still gets excited at the start of each day and the opportunities it will bring.

Sports never interested me. As a kid growing up outside San Francisco my favorite pastime was the radio. When school got out, I couldn't wait to get home and listen to the shows. Radio was our generation's form of entertainment, whether it was comedy, drama, or shows like *One Man's Family* or *Jack Kirkwood's Breakfast Club*. It fascinated me, as if words were flying through the air and coming through a metal box. And after all these years, it still has a solid grip on me. Comedy shows were my favorite, although I listened to just about anything that came over the airwaves.

As an only child with divorced parents, I lived with my mother, who worked odd jobs in the Bay Area in the catering business. My dad was a housepainter, but having a house painted during the depression was not much of a priority so he also did his share of odd jobs. He owned a bait and bar store at one time where I worked with him during the summers. He'd pour the beer and wine up front and I'd sell tackle and pack bait in the back. I had to get up at four in the morning in order to make the wooden boxes, pack them with ice chips, and put the bait in the boxes to have it ready for the early morning fishermen. After that job I couldn't eat fish for years. I didn't know we were poor. With my radio and comic books, my life was full. It was unusual to have divorced parents back then but they tried to make the situation work and I always felt I had access to both of them.

Not liking sports really put a damper on my high school years; I was never one of the guys, never had a lot of friends. My mom wrote notes to get me out of gym class and sometimes it worked. When it didn't I would be forced to play baseball or soccer or whatever the seasonal sport was, but I never enjoyed it. Besides, I was busy after school with paper routes, selling magazines or cutting lawns trying to make a dollar. But I was a happy kid, I just had other interests that weren't the norm for the popular clique of kids.

During high school World War II was in full swing and I

wanted to do something to show my support for the troops. Using my limited theatrical skills, I put together my own USO show to entertain the troops in the Bay Area. I did comedy and magic and was also the emcee. Being good wasn't all that important, because the troops were so appreciative of any form of entertainment. They seemed to enjoy it but probably not as much as I loved doing it.

My senior year of high school I landed a job at a local radio station, one of the first in our area to switch to the music format. I worked in the record library selecting albums, 78s in those days, from the shelf; in the afternoon I hosted my own show, *The Rhythm Review*. The manager of the station took an interest in my future, convincing me to go to college. My mother sold our house to help pay the tuition. The College of the Pacific accepted me as radio major on a work-study basis. To fulfill my job requirements, I became the announcer for a local baseball team. That's the closest to sports I ever got. Other job responsibilities included organizing the rallies and bonfires for the huge sum of fifty cents an hour. The best job, though, was working at the two campus radio stations.

By my junior year in college, 1948, I quit school and entered the job market. The war had ended and I knew jobs would be scarce but I had experience on my side and soon had a job selling radio time. My manager was a great guy who really knew how to motivate people. He made work fun. A few years into my job, a fellow I'd known at college approached me with a new job offer to go to New York and start up a one-man operation selling radio time. Without even the blink of an eye, I was on a plane to New York, not knowing a soul and not having a penny in my pocket. To this day, it was the best decision I ever made. My career can be summed up in less than a minute: worked for a radio station in high school, majored in radio at college, met a fellow who asked me to join him in the radio sales business, moved to New York, and been here ever since. Along the way, that one-man operation became the largest national radio sales company in America, employing 650 people worldwide. The end.

When I got to New York, I set up an office and spent my days walking up and down the streets knocking on doors and selling. It was hard work, but I loved it; it didn't feel like work. Never exercised, unless you consider walking the streets of New York City exercise. Never played tennis, hit the golf ball, or wanted to. The only physical form of exercise I ever thought of doing was taking tap dance lessons, but that was a secret I never shared with anyone until I was forty-nine years old.

Why tap dancing? Growing up watching Fred Astaire, Gene Kelly, and Donald O'Connor in the movies. I always wanted to be able to dance like them. They were the greatest dancers of their time. Tap dancing looked like fun and something that anyone could do. I made a promise to myself that someday I would take tap, but never got around to it. When I was forty-nine, I held a time management seminar at my company and hired Allan Lakin, who wrote *How to Get Control of Your Time and Your Life,* to run the seminar. One of the exercises he conducted was to close our eyes, relax, and imagine that we had all the time in the world to do whatever we really wanted to do and then write down that one thing. I wrote "learn to tap dance." Lakin summed up the exercise by saying if you don't have the time to do what you really want to do, why are you doing all these other stupid things you don't like all day? He made an impact on me and that thought stayed in my mind.

A few weeks later it was my birthday and I received a book and a set of six tap dance lessons from my employees. The author of the book, Bob Audy, was regarded as the best tap dance teacher in the world. His clients included Shirley MacLaine, Ben Vereen, Joel Grey and John Travolta. As fate was with me, he was also located in New York, not far from my office, so I immediately went out and signed up for his class and that's where I spent my lunch hour. Tap dancing was much more difficult than I ever imagined; far more difficult than selling radio advertising. At first I felt like I had two left feet and no coordination at all. But the beauty of tap is in its joyous form and happy tempo. You can't help but feel good after a lesson. It was fun and I loved it. The exercise part of it was just a by-product, but a healthy one. The aerobic benefits are incredible. Not that I was out of shape, but I wasn't in shape either. After the six lessons were over, I was hooked and kept up the lessons going two or three times a week. After doing this for quite a while, I calculated the number of hours spent commuting to the studio, plus the hour lesson, and it totaled about 156 hours out of my life. That's four weeks of work a year. So it was a business-driven decision to build my own studio at the office; much more efficient and cost effective than taking the cabs and wasting all that work time. Call it phony logic or whatever, I love having the studio, and it is in use all day. As an owner and manager, I've always believed that employees should have as much fun as the boss, so the studio is available free of charge to anyone who wants to take tap. The next best thing to happen was that Bob closed his own studio and came to work full time for me.

Over the years the studio has grown to include not only tap

but also jazz, ballroom dancing, aerobic workouts, and stretching exercises. It took on a life of its own. Employees took such an interest in the dancing aspect that we decided to put on a holiday revue at our year-end party that has evolved to the point where we have a waiting list for participation. Bob, who is not only a professional dancer but a choreographer as well, directs the show. Complete with costumes, music, special lighting, and three months of rehearsals, it is the most talked-about event of the year.

When I am tap dancing, I don't think of anything else in the world. It takes away all stress. Tap absolutely demands that you relax and keep a smile on your face. Even when you make a mistake, and I make plenty, you crack up with laughter. And in a full classroom, you can actually hear the mistakes, so everyone laughs. After making a mistake I just listen to the music, count out the steps, take a deep breath, and begin again. The concentration is very demanding, and if my mind starts to wander back to business I'll find myself a few steps behind everyone else. Tap dancing is very aerobic and is also highly mathematical. I have to employ both sides of my brain when tapping or I mess up. Everything is done in units of eight. It is very artistic and for someone like me who never enjoyed any kind of sport, this is my idea of physical activity. Regardless of age, sex, or physical shape, there is nothing to fear in tap. You can't fall, there's no jumping so basically you never hurt yourself, and the positive side effects include improved muscle tone in the legs and better posture. And if you think of yourself as uncoordinated, tap can improve your coordination. It will teach you a vocabulary of sounds and counting; with concentration you can build on those sounds and improve. The satisfaction is immediate as well as gratifying.

I've always believed that anything you can imagine you can do, you can. My parents always told me that, and I always believed them. There are so many opportunities out there for anyone who wants to go after them. I don't view my ten-hour days as work. There are mornings when I am up at 4:30, attend breakfast meetings, go through the day, attend a function at night and finally get to bed at 11 P.M. I couldn't do that every morning, but if I can't sleep I will sit at the computer and send e-mails. I have a reputation for working all the time, but it's all a mind-set. I'm not that different from anyone else, didn't have any breaks in life. Short of any critical illness, people have to learn to get on with their lives and go after what they want. It's that simple. I still attend my high school reunions. Most of the people have led interesting lives and have something to share, to offer in conversation. But there are always one or two high school jocks who are still reliving that one fabulous play they made and consider it the best time of their life. They let life pass them by and that's unfortunate. They have nothing to look forward to. You have to learn to look forward to change. I get excited every day over what prospects I may find.

My wife and I have been married for fifty years, have five children and sixteen grandchildren. All my children are associated with the radio business. We also have an intern program for juniors in college and we let the interns stay in our house. I get a kick out of them and it allows me to stay in touch with the trends of the younger kids. We watch TV together and I can tell you what's happening on *Ally McBeal*. I don't want to just hang out with people my age. I feel that if you want to keep growing mentally as well as being physically fit, you have to surround yourself with people who are interesting and engaging and will challenge you with new ideas and concepts.

I'm healthy, I'm active in my field and I have plans for the future. I get a checkup every year. In fact, I tend to be a bit of a worrier about my health. If you tell me your neighbor has a brain tumor, I'll get a checkup. My doctor says not to bother him with this nonsense. But think about it: How many people do you know who died of an illness and the doctor said, "If only we'd caught it earlier"? I'm making sure my doctor catches whatever it is early enough, so I get the checkup.

Retirement plans are not in my near future. Why should I select a successor when I'm not ready to retire? The right person selected today may not be the right person five years from now. But between you and me, I am never going to retire; couldn't bear to leave my tap studio. Nothing short of retirement, and not even then, will stop me from putting on my tap shoes and tapping away all my problems.

ROAD WARRIOR

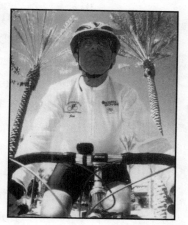

JAMES HOUSE

Date of birth: 4-27-25

RESIDENCE: Sun City Grand, Arizona

"When I see an adult on a bicycle, I do not despair for the future of the human race." —H.G. Wells

Jim was referred to me through the Huntsman World Senior Games staff. At first I didn't think I should interview him, because he had been active in sports most of his life and I was looking for late bloomers. Jim may have been active, but he wasn't healthy. He convinced me that he had a very serious and important message to deliver, so we continued the interview. Here is what Jim wrote me after reviewing his chapter: "Miss Gail, when someone reads about me, I not only want them to note that I changed my entire outlook on life by becoming health conscious, but also want to give them a guide to what they can do to achieve the same results. No matter how many assets you have, it is very difficult to be happy if you are not healthy. Please note the importance of resting heart rate, blood pressure, blood lipids, percent of body fat, body-mass index and keeping them in the correct range. Daily aerobic exercise is the best medicine in the world."

Although I exercised in my middle years, dabbling in running and tennis, I never did a good job of it. Wasn't in good shape, was overweight, and yet there I was playing tennis and pounding the roads. Not having good eating habits also meant my cholesterol was high. I was the perfect heart attack poster boy. You've all seen me, or someone like me: I'm the guy running or playing tennis thinking I'm a great athlete but in reality I was not doing myself any favors. But let me start at the beginning.

I grew up in Big Rapids, Michigan, delivered by a doctor who arrived just in time in a horse and buggy. The population of our town was five thousand, if you counted the chickens, dogs, and horses. During the summers I lived with my grandfather on his farm and did all sorts of chores. I was up before dawn and in bed after dark. It was hard work. And for all my efforts, he paid he me seventy-five dollars for the entire summer. When the depression came, our family suffered but we were better off then most. I thought we were rich compared to other families who didn't have clothes or food. My father never lost his job. But most of my adult life, I've suffered from the Depression Disease, always counting pennies and never wasting food. At mealtime, I would put only one thing at a time on my plate. The ultimate symptom of the Depression Disease is that you become so damn cheap throughout your life, afraid to spend any money even if you have enough to be comfortable. You don't throw out socks with holes because they're still good. You eat food you don't even like because it's there. That type of mentality isn't healthy, and it took me a while to overcome it.

When the war came, I was eighteen and enlisted in the army air force and became a bombardier. Flew a lot but was lucky enough to escape without a scar on me. I also served two and a half years in Korea. I married my childhood sweetheart before I went to war and came home to settle down and go to college. If it weren't for the GI Bill there'd be no college, because I couldn't afford it. The marriage didn't last, but I did graduate and continued on for a master's degree. We were way too young and our marriage, like most wartime rushed nuptials, was doomed from the beginning. Eventually, at thirty-three, I married a woman with three children and we quickly added one more. This time, it worked.

As far as sports, I always ran for fun. Lettered in track in high school. Stopped for a while during the war and college. Those five years of college at Michigan State were tough. I wasn't too smart and it was hard work. Bad combination. Plus my chosen field, chemical engineering, was demanding. Michigan State is a very large campus and since we couldn't even think of buying a car, I bought a cheapo bike to get around to classes. When I finished school, I was finished with that bike for good. After graduation I got a job and moved to Ohio.

The wife, the kids, and I settled down in Ohio. I started to pick up running again at thirty-five, but it was very unstructured. If it rained, I didn't go out. If I didn't feel like it, I didn't go out. No schedule, no running calendar. I just ran for fun. All through this period I was overweight and never bothered with medical checkups. Junk food was my favorite meal, especially doughnuts and chocolate. I ate everything in sight but the squeal out of the pig. As a kid back on the farm, we butchered our own meats, and the slabs of bacon we cut for meals were pure fat. It was good! Nobody ever talked of cholesterol levels or body-fat percentage. I didn't know if it should be 90 or 19. My wife worked at the University of Dayton and they offered a health program for their employees and families. She went and thought it would be good for me, so I went reluctantly. Actually, I was dragged along. They called it a Wellness Program, headed by university doctors. When I finally got a check-up, my doctor told me all the bad news: I was overweight with a high cholesterol count. I listened, but continued to gain weight. The doctor had a nice bedside manner when I started on the Wellness Program, but when I continued to gain weight he got mean. Told me I could be his poster boy for a heart attack ad. Told me I was living on borrowed time. This time I listened and did something about it. He scared me. I was fifty years old and failing all the medical tests. Time to change.

Retiring at sixty-two, we moved to Arizona. I started playing more tennis, although my knees bothered me from my previous years of activities. I played on hard court surfaces; they don't usually use clay courts in Arizona, due to the heat and low humidity. More bad news for my knees. My knees got so bad I couldn't roll over in bed at night without feeling excruciating pain. I was in a bad way; I didn't want to give up tennis because I knew my weight would balloon again, but yet the pain was unbearable. Finally I went for a consultation on knee surgery. The doctors advised against it. They felt I'd just wear them out again, and they also weren't too high on going through surgery just so I could play tennis. I was sixty-five at the time and they talked me out it. So now what was I do to? Can't play tennis, can't run, and can't even walk. I was one sad kid.

I decided to go back to biking. Hadn't been on one since my college days, but there in the garage was my daughter's bike, a little lady's pink three-speed with big balloon tires. So I hopped on and took a ride. Went grocery shopping. Did it early in the morning so there wouldn't be any traffic and also so no one would see me. Riding a bike is like swimming. Once you know how, you just get right back into it. I knew I needed the exercise and couldn't just sit around with my finger up my ear. Also, I wanted to exercise. Missed it. Eventually I did go out and buy my own bike. Met up with a few guys my age who were bikers, and they talked me into riding with them. We were doing fifteen- and twenty-mile rides, which I could handle. One day as we started out for our ride, they forgot to tell me that ride would be fifty miles! I thought I'd die. But I did it. It was extremely tough. I had a terrible time with the breathing. Running is aerobic but tennis isn't. In tennis you hit the ball for a while, it goes out of bounds, and you take a break. You hit the ball a few more times, the game is over and you take a break. You serve, and a few more bang, bang, bangs, the point is over, and you take a break. Especially in doubles. One guy hits the ball while the other one stands there. I lost a lot of my endurance playing tennis. Biking is hard work. It took me six months to work up to a decent ride. And I went out every day. This was my new job and I wanted to do well.

The next thing they talked me into was doing the time trials for the Arizona Senior Olympics. It was being held right in our neighborhood so I thought, Why not? Surprisingly, I came in first in my age group. I don't know why I did so well, except for the fact that I had built up my endurance. But even with that, it was very tough. I know I sounded, and looked, like I was going to die. The crowd expected me to just tip over and die. It was a very exciting day. That was ten years ago and it changed my life. At sixty-five, I discovered bike racing and have been going strong ever since. And about those knees: I never have pain. In biking there's no impact and no lateral movement of the leg to cause the pain that the running and tennis brought on. I'm a new man.

I can't say enough for how exercise has saved my life. It keeps my cholesterol down, my body fat down, my weight down—and I eat better. Actually, I eat like a pig because I burn it all off. When I go for my annual medical checkups, I get a pat on the back for good behavior instead of a kick in the butt for screwing up. Also sleep soundly every night, a good solid eight hours, and wake up rarin' to go. Everything stays dandy! And even if I do overeat, which usually happens around Christmastime, and put on a few extra pounds that just hang there, I know I'll burn them off once I'm back on the bike. It's not the same kind of weight gain as the three-hundred-pound person who can't stop eating the box of chocolates and has no outlet to lose it. I also get lots of positive reinforcement not only from the doctors, my family and friends, but also from the people I meet at the race events. They see a seventy-five-year-old man out there breaking records and winning medals and they like it. I like it.

The mental aspects of exercise are also very important. First of all, your friends tend to be just like you; dedicated to exercise and just wanting to have fun. A healthy, happy bunch of people, even if some of us have cancer or heart disease or other ailments. We don't depend on alcohol or drugs or that five o'clock cocktail to get through the day. It's a healthy mode. We can't wait for the next race, not the next drink. We meet every morning for a ride and there's no pressure if you don't show up. We make sure everyone gets home safely. It's a nice group of people, all doers.

My routine doesn't vary much: thirty miles a day unless I have a race coming up, then I'll cut down on the mileage the day before. I'm usually up anytime between 3:30 and 5 A.M. to get in my breakfast, stretching and then gear up for a thirty-to-forty-mile bike ride. The early-morning hours are a great way to beat the Arizona heat. No way would I choose to do my ride at noon when the temperature is already soaring. On alternating days I do an hour-long workout with weights. And just so you don't think I'm a fanatic, I do stay away from mountain biking. I have enough trouble falling down on nice smooth surfaces; I'm not interested in going down in the cactus and stones. My children, who range in age from thirty-five to fifty, worry about me but I worry more about them, because they're all couch potatoes.

I do about twelve thousand miles a year, give or take a few hundred. My favorite sweatshirt is emblazoned with the motto, NEVER UNDERESTIMATE THE POWER OF AGE. I don't look my age, and I certainly never did act my age. I know I'm not twenty-one, but I don't feel seventy-five. Actually, for most of my life people thought I was older than my age due to the fact my hair turned completely white in the war. Now I am regressing. I wear a sign on my back that reads, YOU HAVE BEEN PASSED BY A 75-YEAR OLD. After the race they come up to me and say, "How come you wear that sign when you're not that old?" Other people say, "When I grow up I want to be like you." I get a lot of younger guys in my riding area that come out on a Saturday morning and try to beat me. I call them the Saturday Warriors. We have a nice give and take and they usually end up complimenting me and telling me I am an inspiration. That feels good.

I don't pay attention to my times anymore. People always ask, "Did you come in first?" I don't always win, but I hate to lose! I came in second four times in a row in a meet this spring and that hurt. My favorite rides are the time trials that test my experience and endurance. It's the challenge, I guess. I also get to put my biking to good use as a fund-raising participant for charities. In 1998 I rode 504 miles across Arizona to raise money for the purchase of bicycle helmets for my area's elementary school third-graders. I did it with a partner, Kathy Wenzlau, and we had a thrilling adventure. We rode from the Utah boarder to the Mexico border in Nogales, putting in about a hundred miles per day. The winds were a big factor and at times I thought I'd be swept into the Grand Canyon. The scenery was breathtaking. And thank goodness for the support crew that followed us, like the massage therapist who brought our muscles back to life at the end of each day! Corporations also got into the act, such as Prudential and Del Webb Corporation. Another charity event was a seventy-mile fundraiser for juvenile diabetes. I placed seventieth overall in a field of 277 of all age categories and took first place in the over-seventy division and tied for first place in the over-sixty age division. Not bad for a latecomer. Del Webb, the owner of the community, usually covers my normal race and travel expenses. He built the first age-restricted adult community here in Sun City and is now opening up others all over the country. I'm one of his poster boys! He keeps me outfitted in shirts and jackets that advertise Del Webb. The press loves me because I am an active senior, but I always try to use them to get the message out that we are leading vital, exciting, healthy lives that parallel or even surpass our lives prior to retirement.

I never miss an opportunity to encourage others to be active. It's fun and it keeps you healthy. If I can get anyone to wiggle, whether they are five or eighty-five—even just a little—then I've put some sunshine in their lives.

THE FIFTH AVENUE MASTERS MILE MAN

SIDNEY HOWARD

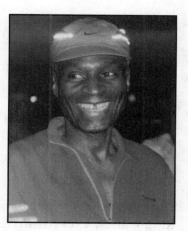

Date of birth: 2-6-39

Residence: Plainfield, New Jersey

"The idea is to die young as late as possible."
—Ashley Montagu

The night Sid came to my house for our interview was also the night of the World Series game when the Yankees won the title. Bad choice in scheduling for me, as Sid kept checking the score. Little did I realize what an impact baseball had had on his life. A high school dropout, married and a father at eighteen—life was hard for this once aspiring high school track star. But Sid persevered and worked hard, opened his own business, stayed married, and raised six kids. He picked up running again at forty to convince his kids that he wasn't old, and the exercise turned out to be the catalyst that got him through some difficult times and will continue to carry this world-record holder into old age. Also got his college degree at age fifty-nine to prove to his grandchildren that anything in life is possible. Describing himself as simple and boring, Sid is anything but.

When I was a kid, I didn't bother much with school subjects. It wasn't until I was eight years old that Jackie Robinson taught me to appreciate reading and love baseball.

My dad and I were big-time baseball fans and spent hours listening to the games on the radio. The Dodgers, the Yankees, the Giants—I knew their names and team numbers by heart. When Jackie Robinson entered the scene, I was totally blown away. The first black player in professional baseball impacted my entire family. I'd see his picture in the sports pages and want to know everything it said about him. That was my impetus to learn how to read. From that encounter I went on to devour the sports section of the *Daily News*. Before too long I knew everything there was to know about baseball. My father brought me around to his pals and had me quote all the batting averages for the Dodgers. Ty Cobb's batting average at the time was .367. It's funny how I could retain any information that had to do with baseball, but nothing to do with fractions; couldn't even do a simple pie chart. I could tell you that a batter was hitting .250 but couldn't figure that was the same as 25 percent, or a quarter of a hundred. This inability to concentrate on numbers caught up with me and eventually got me kicked out of high school.

There were ten kids in my family, five boys and five girls. It was a crowded house. I never slept in bed alone until I joined the air force at seventeen. My younger sister was the only one of us to graduate from high school. My parents had migrated up from Georgia looking for work and brought with them their southern heritage. To tell you the truth, I don't think either of my parents ever attended school. We were very poor, but no matter how little we ate during the week, Sunday morning was a down-home southern feast: grits, biscuits, corn bread, chicken, collard greens, enough food to stuff us for the day. Both my parents worked long hours in the factories, so we had to look after one another. It was understood that the older ones looked after the younger ones. When my parents were home, they were strict disciplinarians. No one dared cross them or disobey. The beatings weren't worth it. We soon learned not to repeat something that displeased my dad.

Baseball and the radio dominated our lives. After school, I'd race home to listen to the *Green Hornet* or the *Fat Man Show*. I was totally absorbed into the radio. It took me away to the extent that I felt I was in the studio with the Fat Man. They were my heroes, along with Jackie and Ty and the other players. When Bobby Thompson of the New York Giants hit the home run in 1951 at the playoff game, the Shot Heard Round the World, and eliminated the Dodgers from the World Series I felt like I lost a kin. My father went into mourning. It was like the air was let out of the room. Baseball was my life. I even dreamed of being a professional ball player but was afraid of the ball.

I guess you could say I was the typical class clown in high school. Never took it seriously. A star on the cross-country team, I thought that my status would spare me from learning simple fractions. I thought the coach would pull rank for his top-flight runner. But when I failed math and wood shop, I was thrown off the team. All I had to do was go to summer school to graduate, but I didn't. Instead, I quit school. Looking back, it was the worst decision I ever made. I decided to join the air force; my father tried to talk me out of it. At first he refused to sign the enlistment papers, but he got so mad at me for being pigheaded he signed in the end. I entered the air force at seventten and came out at twenty-one. I grew up fast during those four years. Had to. I became a husband and father along the way after managing to get my high school girlfriend pregnant before I left for the air force.

We didn't plan on this, as she was only sixteen. It was the very first time we had intimate relations and three months later she announced she was pregnant. But I did the right thing by her; we got married and she had a healthy baby boy. Then we went on to have five more babies. We were babies having babies. I wasn't even shaving yet and had a son! But I have to believe that the Lord looks after fools and babies, and we qualified in both categories. Most stories that begin this way don't have happy endings, but ours did. We stayed married for thirty-nine years, until she passed away from heart disease complications two years ago.

While in the air force, I received my high school equivalency degree. Meantime, my wife finished her high school degree at night school while her parents helped out with the baby. By the time I got out of the air force at twenty-one, we had four kids. When I landed a job as a copy machine operator for a hundred dollars a week, we were able to move into the projects paying sixty dollars a month rent. For ten years we worked hard, trying to save money and raise the kids the best way we knew how. There was no time or money to do anything recreational. I hadn't run since high school, didn't even think about it. For four years I never took a day off, never had a sick day. It was work, work, and more work. In 1970, when I was thirty-one years old, I got a new job as a delivery man, making an astounding $125 a week. My boss trusted me and allowed me to take the truck home on weekends and moonlight on my own for delivery jobs. This brought in even more money. After a month my boss gave me permission to go into business for myself, as long as I agreed to pay him a commission. He set me up with a great client that I kept for years. Even though I didn't have to keep paying him a commission,

I did so for eleven years even without a contract. The way I figured, I wouldn't be in business without him, so I never minded. Over the years, the business grew from $125 a week to $4,000 a month. Thirty years later I'm still in my own business, employing up to twenty-eight people.

Along the way of working too hard and too long and raising five kids, I became a vegetarian. At first I did it as a goof because my older brothers wanted to try it out and I went along for the ride. Three weeks later they reverted back to meat eaters, but I stayed a strict vegetarian. I do think it has made a positive effect on my health. And I'm sure that if my wife shared just a bit of my diet she'd be alive today. She'd make tofu for me then sit down to McDonald's. She never bought in to the theory that you are what you eat. Beans and rice may be boring, but they sure do add up to a better diet than saturated fats. When I go grocery shopping, before I buy anything I ask myself, "Is that good for me? Is that food going to benefit me in any way?" If the answer is no, I pass it by. I've also heard there's a study—unfounded of course—that vegetarians don't beat their wives. We are very peaceful people.

In 1974, when I was thirty-five, one of my clients (who was a copy-editor for a well known publishing house) was responsible for planting the seeds that got me to college. Every week when I went to her house to pick up the manuscripts, she'd have me in for tea while she finished her work. We got to be friends and when she learned I didn't go to college, she made it her goal to convince me to go. My tuition was still guaranteed under the GI bill, even twelve years later, so I decided to attend night school. My motivation at the time wasn't to better myself; it was to use the money I was entitled to. Heck, why not? If the government wants to send me to school, I'll

go. However, after two years the money was used up, but I
continued on my own. I guess I was kind of a late bloomer. I
took psychology, sociology, anything that sounded interesting
and had to do with people. My oldest son was sixteen at the
time and we'd do homework together. It was a shock to me
how much I enjoyed learning. For eight years I attended
night school, thenI just quit. I'd had enough and needed a
break. I didn't intend for that break to last nine years, but just
when I was thinking of never going back I found out that if
you abstained from classes for more than ten years all the
hard-earned credits would be lost. Realizing that college was
a good thing for me, I re-enrolled. Something clicked inside
me and I realized just how much that college degree meant to
me. From 1991 to 1998 I was back at night school earning
every hour that went into my diploma. I loved the class
dynamics and it never bothered me that I was by far the oldest in the class. In fact, it made me realize that I did have
something to offer, that my life had been rich with opportunities in many ways. I also wanted to show my grandchildren
that anything is possible if you want it badly enough. And on
commencement day, nothing in my life to date compared
with graduating from college. All the races in the world, all
the medals I've won could never equal the accomplishment of
getting my degree.

When I was just about forty years old, my son mentioned a
mile race that was being sponsored in town. He said, "Dad,
there's a race for old guys like you at the high school." I hadn't
run in twenty-three years, never even gave it a thought. But
something way back inside me triggered my old glory days on
the track and my love of running poured out and I became
determined to run that race. I trained hard for three weeks

and won the race! My kids were shocked, couldn't believe their old man could run so fast. I didn't even own a pair of running shoes; I ran in a pair of old track shoes. A new world opened up for me and running came back to my life like an old friend. Someone mentioned the New York City Marathon, which I had never even heard of, but it sounded like a good challenge. Three months later I ran the 26.2 miles in 3:02. I never knew I had it in me. Looking back on my high school track days, I guess I just never realized my full potential. And perhaps that was a good thing, because I probably would have burned out early. During the next five years I ran nine marathons with a personal best time of 2:46:27. But marathons are too hard and I gave them up. The training takes too much time. During these years of rediscovering running, I was juggling the kids, my wife's early stages of heart disease, working all day, and attending school at night. This may sound crazy, but running was the catalyst for everything. Running gave me the energy to get through the rest of the day. The day started at five-thirty in the morning with a run before going to work and the day just seemed to glide by. It became important to me. I'd try to get my kids to run by bribing them, but even money couldn't get them out the door. They'd come up with imaginary aches and pains in their ankles and knees and feign a few limps. They taught me a valuable lesson: If you don't want to do it for yourself, you won't do it at all.

After giving up marathons I switched to track and ran shorter distances of three- to six-mile races. Missing the competition and camaraderie of a team, I joined the Central Park Track Club, and that opened up my career. When the New York Road Runners Club started the Fifth Avenue Mile in

1983—a very prestigious run that attracts the top talent—I entered. It's my favorite race and I believe I am the only masters runner who has run that event every year. My efforts finally paid off and in 1999, at age sixty, I won my division. I never thought I could run this fast. And the funny thing is I keep getting faster! My times have improved over the past five years. That may sound crazy, but runners are not normal people. We have to be a bit nuts to do what we do.

Turning sixty has been the best year of my life. Not only did I get to enter a new age division in racing, but my accomplishments have been better than I ever wished for. I hold the world record for the indoor 800-meter masters championships and the American masters record for the outdoor 800 meters.

You know, I'm just a simple boring guy. I eat, run, work, sleep, in that order. When my wife was sick, I took care of her the best way I could. It was time consuming, an act of love and devotion, but in a way it left me with little time to think about the suffering and devastation it placed on us. Now I live alone and really miss her. The kids are out of the house and have busy lives of their own. My days are still filled with morning runs; then I'm out the door to work till late in the evening and sometimes weekend work as well. When I want to relax and have fun, I go dancing. My kids and grandkids are a big part of my life because I know how important family ties are. As a kid I visited my grandfather every weekend. He lived to be a hundred and was still sharp as a tack. We had great times together. Sometimes we'd team up and goof on my father, who was very religious and didn't take well to remarks against his beliefs. My grandfather loved to tease him and would say things like, "Hey Sid, do you think you can really get into heaven without being baptized?" My father always took the bait and we'd be in for some heated rounds. My own father died before my grandfather. Even though Jackie Robinson was my first hero, my dad was my second. And after he died, my grandfather took his place. He was a gift to me and I returned that gift by spending my weekends with him. I also regularly visited my aunt when she was in a nursing home. I've always believed that you have to be a giver in order to receive. My kids have learned from watching me and put aside time to spend time with their families.

At sixty, I don't consider myself old. It's mind over matter: If you don't mind, it doesn't matter. Exercise has helped me formulate my thoughts on aging, and I have come to the conclusion that most of the ailments associated with aging can be prevented with proper diet and exercise. I used to be a smoker. Started smoking when I saw all the baseball players puffing away on their Lucky Strikes. That was my brand, because I saw it advertised at the Dodgers games. And when I was in the air force, you could always get free time by asking for a cigarette break. I smoked for twelve years and then quit when I decided to get healthy. It was a very hard thing to do, but I've never picked up a cigarette since. It all goes along with my theory that you can do anything you want if you have the discipline and the desire.

You can be healthy at any age if you make the effort. Of course it's easier if you have a good foundation, but healthy habits can start at any age and still show benefits. And you don't have to run marathons to be fit. Walk upstairs instead of taking an elevator. Walk a few blocks instead of taking a cab or subway. It's all in the discipline.

My goal is to not only reach one hundred years old, but to

set the new age-group records for running the mile, three-mile, and maybe even the five-mile. I also plan to be self-sufficient, still drive my own car, dress myself and cook for myself. If I can't have a quality life I don't care much about the quantity. Want to place a bet I make it?

THE KEY TO LONGEVITY IS ACTIVITY

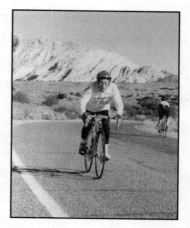

RALPH HOYLE

Date of birth: 12-30-09

Residence: Rexford, New York

> "With years a richer life begins, the spirit mellows:
> Ripe age gives tone to violins, wine and good fellows."
> —John Townsend Trowbridge

This over-ninety athlete has been breaking records in many sporting events since he started competing at seventy-five. Picking up sports to help fill the loneliness after his wife of fifty-eight years passed away, Hoyle turned out to be a natural. He attributes some of his stamina to eating a diet of organic produce since the 1940s. He describes himself as a tough competitor with a heart of gold; the ladies especially love Ralph for his smooth moves on the dance floor. In his first triathlon at the age of eighty-one, he separated his shoulder during the cycling event but got right back on the bike and finished. That's how Ralph lives his life: He never gives up and doesn't show any signs of stopping. He wants to be a role model and prove through his own activities that it's never too late to start something new.

I guess you could call me a late bloomer; I didn't start competing in sports till I was seventy-five years old. Now I can do up to fifty miles on the bike and am working my way up to a hundred. I'm not there yet, but I've got time. I go out ball-room dancing four, sometimes seven nights a week till one in the morning. After dancing we go out for breakfast. The next day I'm a bit tired and tend to sleep later than normal, per-haps till around eleven.

No one in my family was athletic. We were definitely not the active types. My father was a professional singer, but none of us could sing either. Born in Woonsocket, Rhode Island, I came to New York in 1929 to work for the General Electric company. I worked for them on different jobs during my tenure in research and also became a model maker. I also worked on the early jet engine systems and rocket motors. Flying fascinated me. In the 1920s, barnstorming was the big aerial adventure. In the early thirties in California I had the opportunity to go up in a Ford trimotor plane to see the city of Los Angeles from the air. I was always very creative and was good at using my hands. I like to keep busy. During the war I taught the women how to work the machines at the fac-tory while the men were away fighting. I taught all the "Rosie the Riveters." I never did get to serve, as my job was listed as too important to go overseas.

During the depression I was laid off in 1933 and hitch-hiked to California. It was a great experience and along the way I got to see all kinds of sights and even visited the Chicago World's Fair. When I arrived in Los Angeles, jobs were scarce, but I looked up a former boss of mine from the J.J. Newbury store where I'd worked in New England. I was fired from that job, but it wasn't really my fault and I main-tained a good relationship with the boss. All I wanted was enough money for bus fare back home. It was almost impossi-ble to hitchhike going back East; no one drove in that direction. I pleaded with my former boss; told him I'd do any job they needed. What they really needed was someone to do window displays. The boss said, "Son, if you can trim our window at the corner of Hollywood and Vine and catch attention, you've got the job." I spent two days creating a great display using dishes and glassware stacked on a golden riser trimmed with doilies and got the job. I became their main trouble-shooter at all the area stores doing window displays and anything else they needed. After a year I was fired. Seems Newbury's had a rule stating if you were ever fired from one store you couldn't work for the company again. I was disappointed because they were just about to promote me to manager, but as I tell my granddaughter, you can't worry about disappointment. You never know what other doors of opportunity await you.

I decided I'd had enough of California and hopped a bus to Dallas. Stayed there four months and decided I didn't like it, but I had to stay long enough to earn my bus fare the rest of the way home. Bus fare was twenty-eight dollars from Dallas to Boston. Back in Rhode Island I went to work for General Electric again. I was trying to date a girl in the office but she only dated Jewish fellows, so she fixed me up with her girlfriend, May. That first date was June 6, 1936, and we were married the following February. We had one child of our own and then adopted a child. Our younger daughter, who is a nurse, now lives with me. After my wife died she said, "Dad, I don't want you to ever worry about living alone or taking care of yourself. When you need me, just call."

Besides our two daughters, we were also foster parents to three boys. The youngest boy became so close to us we wanted to adopt him, but his mother didn't want to release him at the time. A few years later when she did, I was suffering from bad health and was in and out of the hospital for months, so we were not in a position to take him. The last boy came from a reform school and he was too incorrigible for us. The middle boy ended up in the hospital due to a lactic intolerance we were not aware of, so I raised goats to provide him with goat's milk. We were living on a farm at the time due to my health. Moving to the farm made all the difference in the world to me; I attribute to the farm life my longevity and good health. I should have been a health food store poster boy. We had an organic garden for fifty-five years and lived off the land. So when the foster child needed goat's milk, it seemed natural to raise the goats. We lived on the farm for nineteen years and then abruptly moved to a mobile home in Glenville, New York. That didn't last long and the next move brought us here to Rexford. When I retired the first time at seventy-one, I took up golf and went back as a per diem doing odd jobs. When I retired for the last time, I got a job at a health food store, which was a wonderful learning experience for me. I now take up to twelve supplements a day, and I feel great.

When I turned seventy-five a senior citizens center opened up in town, and a friend and I decided to check it out. The center was trying to get the seniors interested in the local level of the Senior Olympic trial so I went along and participated, just out of curiosity. I won a few medals and it was definitely fun to see my name in the papers. My friend eventually quit going, but I was hooked, got the bug. My events were biking, swimming, racquetball and table tennis. I held the national record for the eighty-to-eighty-nine age division. I'll never forget my first triathlon event at the age of eighty-one. It wasn't memorable because of my age but because my bicycle brakes jammed and I was thrown over the handlebars, separating my shoulder. Instead of quitting, I got right back on my bike and finished the race. Then there was a minor setback in 1992 when I was hospitalized for an unknown condition, which turned out to be hypoglycemia. Before it was diagnosed I was given the wrong medicine and it darn near killed me. Ended up in a wheelchair for a while but six months later I participated in a race walk.

In 1995, after fifty-eight years of marriage, my wife died of cancer. She had been in the hospital for a while and one day the doctor told me, "Ralph, she will never come out alive." I had been scheduled to participate in the Senior Olympic nationals in San Antonio but didn't want to leave her side. She insisted that I go and four days after I came back she died. I think she hung on just for me, and to see all the medals I won. It's interesting that I won the most medals ever while at San Antonio. She was my inspiration and remains so to this day. Athletics fill up my day now that she is gone. My motivation to continue also comes from the camaraderie of competition; I like to meet and talk to people. Of course I like to do well, but mostly it's for the fun of it. I receive a great deal of satisfaction by being with other members of the senior community at these events. They are my friends. And I get to dance with the ladies afterward. But even when I am not competing, I participate through cheering on the other competitors. That's also important, to make others feel special.

Now that I'm ninety, it's hard to think back why I started competing. I guess I just wanted to get off the couch, have something to do. At eighty-four, I climbed the Corning Tower in Albany, forty-two floors. It's a big event and I finished in fifteen minutes and thirteen seconds. I already have my application in to repeat the event this year. I've already started training on my stepper and at the gym.

In 1998 I had a very serious setback, but not too serious to keep me from competing. I had surgery for colon cancer last January. When I was diagnosed, the doctor wanted to perform the surgery right away but I had a competition coming up so I put it off. The cancer was deeper than expected, so the doctor had to perform a colostomy. That doesn't stop me, though. Doesn't even get in the way. What did cause a major problem was falling off my bike in the last competition and almost cracking my skull. The impact was so severe my skin exploded. I suffered memory loss after the accident, and forgot to pack my belongings when I left the hotel. But then again, at my age I don't know if the memory loss is attributable to the accident or just getting old. Now I have two things to blame when I forget!

This year I spent most of September training for the Senior Games in Orlando. First I went to Denver, Colorado, to visit my fifty-four-year-old girlfriend for a few weeks. She makes sure I get out to see her every two months or so. Then I went on to St. George, Utah, for the World Senior Games and then on to Florida. I take my bike everywhere. I have twenty thousand free miles racked up this year alone from traveling around to my competitions. I still drive when I can, if the distance isn't too great. When I go out dancing, I don't drive home till two in the morning sometimes.

My life philosophy is, "You are never too old to start, you are never too old to set a record and if you can't beat them, outlive them." I belong to U.S. Masters Swimmers and U.S. Masters Biking. It keeps me active, and I enjoy it. I also believe strongly that attitude is everything. Recently a friend of mine said he quit a race because he knew he couldn't win. I told him, "You'll never be a winner if you decide to be a quitter." It's the right attitude that makes you a winner. Never let what you can't do interfere with what you can do. If I can't bike anymore due to my fall, I'll swim. There's always something out there to do. I don't let anything stop me from moving forward. Even these days, when I am in constant pain in my shoulder from the bike fall, I just deal with it. I've also had arthritis pain for years but I just live through it. I will admit the colostomy made me feel old. I used to wear a heart monitor because one of my valves does not operate at 100 percent. According to my monitor charts I wasn't supposed to go over 120, but every time I did my normal exercises I'd be over. Finally my cardiologist told to me throw the damn thing away; I really didn't need it. He said, "When you get tired, quit. If you are tired the next day, slow down until you get your breath back."

The key to my athletic longevity is taking it slow. I do some form of exercise every day, but with a slow, gradual start. If I wake up with stiff muscles, I take a whirlpool at the gym to loosen my legs and arms and get them ready for action. I'm starting to slow down and only exercise three days a week. But every day there is still something to look forward to. I have a lifetime membership in the Holiday Inn Swim Spa near my home and I look forward to a nice soak in the hot tub. Not only does it feel great, but it helps my injuries. I also have a lifetime YMCA membership and recently joined Bally's Gym so I can get a good workout. I try to be an inspiration to the younger people. Sure I have to slow down, stop occasionally and rest, but I always get up and finish whatever it is I'm doing. Right now I am looking forward to climbing those forty-two floors at the Corning Tower. And when my time is up, most likely it will be while I'm on the dance floor. I've had my eye on a new dance partner but she's playing the field so I said the heck with that and got myself another partner. I'm still chasing the ladies at ninety.

When I was in the wheelchair, I had hallucinations. One was so real, I remember it to this day. I went to St. Peter and said, "Are you ready for me?" And he said, " No, go down and talk to the devil and see if he's ready for you." So I went down to see the devil and he came out with his horns and tail and pitchfork and I said, "St. Peter doesn't want me. Are you ready for me yet?" And he said, "No Ralph, you go back up on earth and heckle some of those women you've been bothering these past few years." So now I have the devil's permission to misbehave.

Starting work at age nine and retiring at seventy-one didn't afford a lot of leisure time, so I am definitely having more fun in my second childhood than the first. I try to send a message to people approaching retirement to change their lives, to get more out of life, to let them know they can still achieve goals even though they didn't do so when they were younger. There's more to life than making a living and sitting in a chair.

THE LAST ONE ALIVE WINS

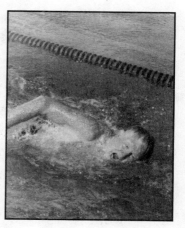

RICHARD KANE

Date of birth: 7-12-11

Residence: Boca Raton, Florida

> **"Age is a matter of feeling, not of years."**
> **—George William Curtis**

Richard grew up swimming in the pristine waters off Staten Island back in the 1920s, but his favorite sport was curtailed while he was stationed in North Africa during the war and then busy raising a family in Virginia. After retiring to Florida, his wife lost a five-year battle to Parkinson's disease. Devastated and neglecting his own health, he knew he had to do something to pull his life together. That something was swimming. At seventy-nine years old Richard dug out his old swim trunks, found a masters swim coach, and turned his life around. Today he has never felt better, or younger. He swims with a pacemaker and still manages to break records in his age group. Exercise saved his life, and every morning he looks forward to a bright future.

Never in my wildest dreams did I ever think I'd be swimming competitively at age eighty-eight. Heck, I didn't even think I'd be alive. It's amazing what swimming has done for a body my age. I wasn't always an athlete but I was always active. Growing up in the Hell's Kitchen area of New York, I had to be on my toes. Luckily, I had a very strict Irish mother who made sure I stayed out of trouble. We didn't know we were poor because everyone was in the same boat. When I wasn't in school or doing odd jobs for extra cash, I was playing in neighborhood pickup baseball or football games. Streets divided the immigrant ethnic groups, each having their own team. Fifty-Fourth Street, where I lived, was mostly Irish with some Italian. The Germans were on Fifty-Sixth, and so forth. We played at Central Park, which was so safe in those days we could be out at midnight without any fear of harm.

My love for swimming came early in life. My family spent summers on Staten Island, where the water was clear and pristine. Mother wanted my older sister Dolly, whom we referred to as pleasingly plump, to lose weight so she gave her swimming lessons. Then my mother, frugal as she was, made Dolly teach the rest of us kids to swim. I spent all summer long in the water. Indoor pools were difficult to come by in New York City so my swimming abruptly ended after summer. When the Knights of Columbus built an indoor pool in Manhattan, I was thrilled. However, they charged fifty cents to get in, which was more money than I had. But I wanted to swim so badly I would scrounge around for a quarter and then hustle a game of handball for the remaining quarter. I was a good player and had a gambler's mentality. I'd lose the first game on purpose and then bet a quarter on the next. Naturally, my victim couldn't resist, so I ended up with the extra quarter and then I could go swim.

My mother wanted us to get a good education that would lead to a well-paying job, so she spent her time looking out our window to see who was driving the cars. She knew that whoever owned cars had good jobs. Right across from our apartment was the jail and courthouse. The court reporters owned some of the cars, so she sent me to secretarial school. Her plan would have worked if I hadn't developed a love for drawing. I was a gifted artist and loved to draw. My mother had me design all the political posters for her bosses at the Democratic club. Without radios or television, the written word was the only form of communicating events. Soon I had the job of drawing all the neighborhood posters. Instead of getting that job as a court reporter, I went on to architectural school. There was no money for school, so I worked as a bank messenger during the day and attended classes at night. That led to a job in Washington, D.C., in 1931 for the Federal Power Commission (now the Department of Energy). I needed to take more classes in math so once again I was working all day and going to school at night. It was a lot of effort. I started swimming at the local YMCA, which was in the process of recruiting a swim team. I lucked out and joined the team. I didn't like the competition at first, but I loved the training. I think I just loved being back in a pool.

Meanwhile, at work everyone was talking about the threat of war, so we were always building contingency plans in case of an attack. I was courting a girl at the time and we were getting pretty close. When the war did come we discussed marriage: Should we or shouldn't we? Already enlisted in the Army, I knew I was going overseas, and Gladys said she wanted more from me than just a letter every week so we got married. We had a brief honeymoon in New York City, which was memorable for the spirit of the people in town. I was always in uniform, and everywhere we went we were never charged a cent. Their hearts seemed to go out to us, the newlyweds who would soon be separated by a war. To this day I have a warm spot in my heart for those folks. Another memorable wartime moment was Christmas Day in Seattle, waiting to be shipped out to Hawaii. Two buddies and I went down to the USO looking for something to do. A woman whose husband was fighting overseas was willing to take us in for Christmas dinner. She and her daughter cooked a beautiful meal. Then the daughter's girlfriend came over to join us and we had a grand time, complete with Christmas presents for us. They even drove us back to the base. When our ship got to Hawaii, we sent them grass skirts as a thank-you. When I think about the war years, I tend to remember the nice moments.

I spent the next four years overseas traveling across North Africa in boxcars called 40-and-8s that were built to carry either forty men or eight horses. Our unit was responsible for mapping Italy, southern France, and North Africa. The last year of the war I was in Hawaii, four stories underground in a pineapple field making maps of the Japanese islands. I was there when the bomb was dropped over Hiroshima.

I left the army in 1945 and went back to my old job in Washington, D.C. Housing was very scarce after the war and we were lucky to find an apartment in Alexandria. Life was busy and there was no time to pick up swimming. Two kids later we needed more room so I borrowed five hundred dollars as a down payment. In 1947 I bought land in Langley, Virginia and designed and built my own house. We couldn't afford a bulldozer so I cleared the land by hand. It took six months just to clear the pine trees for the foundation site. Seven years later, after working on the house nights, weekends, holidays, and vacations, we moved in. Life was beginning to take shape.

As our urban area populated, a few neighbors were interested in starting a community pool. That small spark of an idea turned into the Langley Club, with bathhouse, tennis courts, and pool. It is still operating today. This was heaven for me, as I could finally get back to a regular swim routine doing laps after work. Not satisfied to just lie around swimming, I formed a swim team for the kids and annexed eight other similar clubs in the area to form the Northern Virginia Swimming League. It took up all my free time and nights. My kids were on the team, but I had a sneaking suspicion that the only reason they joined was to attend the Saturday-night swim parties.

In 1972, at the age of sixty-one, I retired. Gladys decided we should move to Florida, where her mother was living and our daughter was attending college. Facing retirement, Gladys made me promise no more swim teams, no coaching, and no long hours of involvement. So instead of swimming, we took up round dancing, which is a form of all couples dancing to the same ballroom steps. When we first started out I only knew a few steps, but we took to it and loved it. We had a group of great friends and we would go round dancing every night. It became our complete exercise and recreation. I still managed a few laps here and there but the dancing took all our time. I've always had a problem with weight, but the dancing kept it off. I loved retirement, loved being with my family in Florida, but the good times were soon to be cut short. Gladys was diagnosed with Parkinson's disease, which she valiantly fought for five years before succumbing to the last dance.

For five years I took care of her the best way I knew how.

She could dance through the Parkinson's, which doesn't affect the brain. She took pills for the shaking, which she timed with her dancing. As soon as the pills took effect she'd glide around the dance floor, beautiful as ever. When the medication wore off, she'd start violently shaking again. Friends who weren't aware of her condition thought she was just tired. I was devastated when she died. I had neglected my own health during those years and was in lousy shape. My weight went up to 240. I failed a routine stress test and the doctor sat me down and told me three things: Lose weight, start exercising, and get out of the house and socialize. I made a resolution not to show up in the obituary column. I spent that Christmas with my son Joseph, who lives in the house we built. Joe was swimming in a masters program and as I watched him do his workout, I thought to myself, Swimming will do it. It's what I've always known, what I've always loved. My son put me in touch with a well-known masters swim coach, Judy Bonning, who turned my life around. Under Judy's careful, almost undivided attention, I accomplished all the doctor's goals. After four months of swimming every day I dropped forty pounds, improved my muscular tone, passed the stress test, and impressed the doctor with my healthy outlook on life. Judy was quite cagey with me at first. When I showed up in my old swim trunks on the first day of our meeting, she took one look at me and said, "Come back wearing a Speedo and we'll see what you can do." I did what she said, but was somewhat embarrassed, as it felt like I wasn't wearing anything at all. She put me through a rigorous routine, but I didn't want competitive swimming and flat-out told her so. But as I said, she could be pretty cagey. She asked me to fill in at a relay one day and that was all it took. I was hooked all over again. In little over a year she transformed me from an out-of-condition seventy-nine-year-old man into a winner of six medals in the 1991 Short Course National Masters Championships. One of those medals was a first place in the 1000-yard freestyle.

Taking the doctor's advice to get out and socialize, I picked up ballroom dancing again and met Irma at a Valentine's dance in 1990. We were married three years later. We're like two teenagers trapped in the bodies of old folks. Actually she's like a youngster to me, as I have sixteen years on her. She's just a kid. When Irma first started swimming with me, she did the "Hudson River breaststroke." She held her head up and it looked as if she was pushing garbage out of the way with her hands. Soon she was into the swim of things, attending meets and competitions with me. She doesn't care much for the competition but she loves the water and traveling to the events. Her medals are for sixth and seventh place but that matters little to us. At our age, the worse you do, the more they clap.

One of my greatest moments was setting a world record in the 200 butterfly at the 1992 international championships in Barbados. I don't set goals for myself so that was a real achievement. When I started swimming masters I did the crawl (freestyle), breaststroke, backstroke, and butterfly. Soon I realized that most of the guys in my age group were good at the first three but no one liked the butterfly. I decided to make that my stroke and it paid off.

In 1994 I fainted in the pool during my workout. I came up sputtering. Lucky for me, a nurse was swimming in the next lane and took me to the hospital. I came home with a pacemaker. At first I was scared to swim again. I was lucky to be swimming at all at age eighty-five and I didn't want to push my luck. What if it stopped working? What if I overexerted myself? But soon I had to take the plunge, and all the worrying was for nothing. I don't even think about. The doctor likes to tease me when I go for checkups and tells me he can't find the darn thing.

I truly think swimming saved my life. After Gladys died I was in such bad shape I could have just given up then. But I didn't. Climbing into the pool was like getting my life back. And then with Irma—well, there's no keeping us down. I swim about an hour almost every day and my weight has been steady at 195. Irma swims on Monday, Tuesday, and Thursday, and Friday gets her hair done. I used to tease her about giving up a day of swimming for her hair, and now she walks in the pool on Fridays! She's a tough one. She beats me in the breaststroke but I'm still trying to catch up.

My whole life has been filled with activity. I've never stopped to sit down and ponder. We still dance and I keep up with my painting. Right now I am teaching my grandchildren to paint. Don't tell Irma I said this, but she was a godsend. My kids tell me how lucky I am to have her. Every day is a great day. Even though we've only been married six years, Irma likes to tell everyone we've been married eighty-five years. That's the combined years we were married to our other spouses and each other.

In my mind I am still young and sometimes that gets me in trouble. When I go to the swim meets, I insist on getting up on the starting blocks. Not many at my age even go near the blocks. They dive in from the pool surface. I just lean on Irma, steady myself, and get up there. When I finally make it up and stand there straight and tall, I say to myself, "You darn fool, someday you're going to fall off this thing and then where will you be?" I did break my pinkie finger last year and it took forever to heal. You know you're old when it takes seven weeks to heal a darn pinkie.

These days I don't have much competition in my eighty-five-to-ninety age division. The only goal I set is to improve my times. There are no rivalries at this age. We're all friendly, and you can usually predict the race before it starts. Masters swimming has made a big splash in the last decade, and I am a big promoter of it. Whether you want to compete or not, I wholeheartedly recommend it. It's a wonderful sport that keeps you fit, is easy on the body and is a great social gathering. You're never too old to swim.

There is no secret to growing old gracefully. I think it's all in the mind-set. I never live in the past, never let unpleasant events pull me down. My outlook is focused on the future and my motto is, "The last one alive wins!" Every morning that I wake, I look forward to another day at the damn pool. That and Irma—but don't tell her—keep me going.

A TOTAL WORKOUT: EXERCISING THE MIND AND BODY

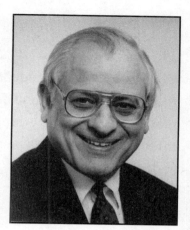

ROBERT KATZ

Date of birth: 12-16-30

Residence: Rockland County, New York

> **"To be seventy years young is sometimes far more
> cheerful and hopeful than to be forty years old."**
> **—Oliver Wendell Holmes**

*Responding to a message I posted on the U.S. Masters Swimming
website, Bob contacted me regarding his late-in-life fitness story, and I
was hooked. We developed quite a lengthy e-mail relationship during
the course of writing his story, as he is passionate about the benefits of
exercise, especially swimming. He started swimming at sixty after
failing a test for the first time: a cholesterol-level reading. His humbling account of seeing himself in a bathing suit after all those lost
years and entering the pool with trepidation will sound all too familiar to those who have been in his shoes. But Bob is not a quitter and
went from a guppie to a shark in months, shedding weight and building endurance and muscle tone along the way. Nowadays he can't
wait to put on a bathing suit and swim more laps.*

My story will probably sound boring but perhaps familiar and can be told in a few seconds. I was a high school athlete (although a better student than athlete), went to college, got married, got a job, had four kids, raised kids (my wife did most of that), and duped myself into thinking that all through those years my calves were still bulging, my abdomen flat as a board, and my thighs rock hard. Turning fifty, I was still in denial about my personal prowess, although I was starting to have trouble walking. Turning 69, I thought doing some mild form of exercise was in order and joined a local pool. Jumped in, swam four feet and collapsed from exhaustion. Now you get the longer version.

I was born in Chicago, had an older brother. We lived a comfortable life. Then the depression hit and my parents lost everything. Then to make my life more difficult my mother developed cancer when I was nine, and since we couldn't afford proper treatment she died a slow death four years later. My life was pretty routine for most kids my age during that time: I played the usual school sports; had a paper route that paid fifteen cents an hour, and was a Boy Scout. Living on the shore of Lake Michigan, we were all were good swimmers and had great times just playing around in the water.

After graduating from high school, I followed my older brother to New York. When my mother died he had taken me under his care like a surrogate parent. He went on to Harvard, but I was having trouble concentrating on what I really wanted to do with my life, so I drifted. My days were spent in the library reading all the philosopher kings and trying to find the meaning of life; my nights were spent at Brooklyn College taking math and physics courses. Studying was the only occupation that kept me going. Eventually I enrolled in a yeshiva seminary and studied Judaism for ten years, becoming an orthodox rabbi. And after thirteen years of night courses I finally graduated from Brooklyn College in 1962.

With such a diverse background, you'd think I'd end up with some fascinating job combining Judaism with math, but at the age of thirty-two my first job was with IBM. For thirty-three years I was the corporate guy with the desk job and occasional travel. Sports had totally disappeared from my life a long time before, replaced with intellectual pursuits. As I mentioned, my physical image of myself never changed from high school. Doesn't matter that over the years I put on weight, increasing from a high school low of 148 to 198. Doesn't matter that I certainly didn't look the same or feel the same. Mentally I was still seventeen. I guess my intellectual pursuits didn't include a reality check of my current physical state.

Retiring from IBM at sixty-three, I wasn't ready to quit working and sit down and get cozy on the couch. Keeping busy keeps me going. My wife didn't want me sitting around all day and my kids didn't want me offering advice all day, either, so I did two things: hit the local campaign trail running for office, and went back to school. Part of politics is getting in shape for all the handshaking so I started to walk around the block. Not too much, just enough to keep me from panting. But I still remember the morning in 1994 when I was running for a bus and sensed my legs weren't working correctly. At sixty-four, I thought it was just another sign of getting old and ignored it. I also ignored the fact that most sixty-four-year-olds don't matriculate back to college. By then my list of degrees included a BA from Brooklyn College in physics, a masters in psychology from the New School, and a doctorate of divinity from the seminary. Being back in school, this time surrounded by kids less than half my age, was a wonderful experience. At first the kids shot me looks as if I was in the wrong place, but over time we got to know and respect each other. I must admit, I went out of my way to meet them. Why not? It was their world I was entering and it was a great experience to learn what they were thinking and how they expressed their views. And this time around I finally learned something hands-on and ended up with an associates degree in LAN (local area networking), which helped land me a civil servant job with the county.

By September 1998, three years into my new job, I still hadn't taken up any exercise and even quit the walking I did during my campaigns. Oh yes, I did pull out an old stationary stepper, but after a few nights it became a clothes rack. One day two posters caught my eye: One was for cholesterol testing, which would be the first test I ever failed in my life; the other was for a fifteen-dollar pass for swimming at the community college pool. Knowing it was time to stop grieving my lost youth and denying my age, I decided to take up swimming. How bad could it be to get in a pool after all those years jumping into Lake Michigan? I was sure it would all come right back to me. The good news was that I still had a bathing suit; although not what you would call stylish, it fit. The bad news was that I had to confront myself in the locker room mirror and realize I had become a fat old geezer. I was mortified.

It was too late to turn back so I sheepishly went out to the pool, headed for the shallow area, and plunged right in for an immediate shock. Why didn't anyone tell me it would be cold as hell! All around me people were swimming like fish and I looked like a beached whale. Too embarrassed to leave without doing anything, I tried out my old backstroke and after four strokes collapsed; I could hardly make it out of the pool. I had no idea I was so badly out of shape. If the cold water wasn't enough of a wake-up call, that certainly was. Humiliated, I headed home.

If I were a quitter, my story would end here, rather unhappily. But I'm not, although I had to think twice about going back. And I did go back again, and again, each time going a little farther. Finally after one month I swam the entire length of the pool. The other swimmers, strangers at first, gave me incredible encouragement. The first few days, as I floundered in the water wondering if there was hope for me, they would tell me what a great job I was doing. No corrections or advice, just pure encouragement. After a while I started to feel comfortable in the water. Their encouragement was a starting point, but what I really needed was technique. I had none. My swimming had been reduced to flapping my arms and legs in the water hoping I moved forward. But thanks to my role models in the lanes next to me, I watched and learned. And then I discovered something that saved my swimming life forever: the U.S. Masters Swimming website. I thought I had died and gone to heaven when I found their discussion forum page. Now I could ask all my questions about form and technique and have pros answer them. One of the self-help tools offered was a total immersion video. After applying what I saw on the video, I was able to cut my stroke count from twenty-seven to sixteen for one pool length by eliminating excess drag and resistance. Thanks to them, a neophyte swimmer was transformed into a fish. Make that a shark.

There have been so many positive benefits added to my life since I started swimming. For one thing, I lost weight. People who hadn't seen me in five months all commented on my new appearance. As one friend put it, "Bob, you lost your fat behind." I took it as a compliment. I have new swim trunks and a Speedo watch just for swimming that tells me more than I will ever need to know, but I wear it proudly. Five months into my venture I can now swim for a solid hour without stopping or becoming fatigued, an accomplishment to be proud of. And I stick to my weekly routine, swimming six days a week in the evening. That's the only time I can fit it in as I still work full time for the county, continue to take more classes at the community college, and manage to keep my wife and kids an active part of my life.

And I have become a health advocate, preaching to my family and friends about the benefits of exercise and trying to get them motivated and moving. Do as I did, I'll say. Unlearn your bad habits and get into a healthy exercise program. They think I'm a born-again Peter Pan.

Too many people fall into the trap of not exercising and create a bumpy rut for themselves. It's obscene and self-serving, a manifestation of greed and a self-defeating philosophy. And it constantly reinforces a bad self-image, which over time creates friction and trouble. If you lose weight, get on an exercise program, keep fit, and keep busy you'll do yourself and others a lot of good. Find out what it is that motivates you in the morning and gets you out of bed.

The greatest satisfaction in life is not winning the lottery or how many orgasms you can have, but to establish a goal and stay dedicated to that goal through hard work and determination. Make every day a challenge. My challenge is to live long enough to attend my grandchildren's weddings. That and swimming more laps.

THE SILVER TENOR

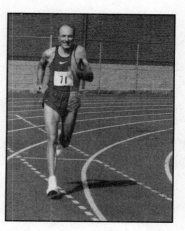

JOHN KESTON

Date of birth: 12-5-24

Residence: McMinnville, Oregon

> "Youth is not a time of life. It is a state of mind . . .
> Live every day of your life as though you expect to live
> forever." —Samuel Ullman

As a teenager John survived the World War II bombings around his native London and enlisted in the air force. When his squadron was sent overseas in Italy, he fell in love with opera. Blessed with a gifted voice, he spent most of his young adult life pursuing a singing and stage career in London and the United States What he didn't realize was that his voice would be an integral part of his becoming a gifted runner later in life. Running his first race at fifty-five, and his first marathon at almost sixty-one, John succeeded in his goal of becoming a starnot only on the stage, but on the track as well. He holds the record as the oldest runner in the world to break three hours in a marathon (2:58:32) which he did at the age of sixty-nine. An internationally acclaimed and respected actor and singer, he appears as Gehn in the CD-ROM computer game Riven. When asked the secret to his running abilities late in life, he sums it all up as his bloody-mindedness. Only a Brit could get away with that, although John became a citizen of the United States in 1995.

In 1942, when I was sixteen years of age, World War II was in its third year. London was being continuously bombed by the German Luftwaffe. Our own home on the outskirts of London had received its share of devastation. The war to a sixteen-year-old was an adventure. I had no regard for my own safety in air raids when the German air force was raining down incendiary bombs to set fire to strategic and even domestic targets. On more than one occasion I extinguished these firebombs, smothering them with sandbags. We were taught that the sandbags should cover one's body when approaching the burning object, because even though the bombs had already ignited, they could explode again to accelerate more destruction.

I was working in an aircraft factory making parts for bomber and fighter planes, which piqued my interest in flying. At sixteen and a half I joined the Royal Air Force, although I had to lie about my age. The legal age to enlist was eighteen, so I forged my documents. I was not allowed to become a pilot because of a hernia problem, but the RAF was desperate for aircraft mechanics so I went to school for eight months at a training facility in Wales. Upon graduation, I was posted to the 603d City of Edinburgh Fighter Squadron. Our Spitfire squadron had fought in the Battle of Britain with distinction. By now the air defense of Britain was basically won, so the unit was sent overseas to serve as air support for Montgomery's campaign against Rommel in the North African desert. We were in a very large convoy of ships; none of us knew the route or our destination. It was somewhere in the middle of the ocean that I was summoned to our commanding officer's cabin and questioned about my true age. The CO had received word from HQ that I was underage. My mother had contacted RAF headquarters and told them I was too young to serve. My CO explained that my mother had been told it was too late; I had already gone. Then my CO commended me for my patriotism.

After the desert campaign ended, my squadron was sent to Italy. While stationed in Naples, I saw my first opera. The tenor was impressive, singing the famous flower song. Fifteen years later I would be singing the same aria, portraying tenor Don José, in Bizet's *Carmen* at Indiana University.

When the war was over, I returned home to London no longer the adventurous teenager but a twenty-one-year-old man with wife, a Maria, whom I had met and married in Naples. There was much rebuilding going on and the ravages of the war were everywhere. Most of the returning soldiers got involved with re-building the bombed-out areas but I wanted a musical career and applied for a British government grant. I had already been accepted at London's Trinity School of Music, but unfortunately there was no money for the performing arts. The government's offer was free tuition to become a bricklayer, carpenter, electrician, etc. So Maria, our baby Anthony, and I returned to Italy where I worked as an interpreter and studied singing, paying for my own lessons. After six months of daily lessons we returned to England.

I had developed a fine tenor voice but, lacking professional experience, needed to sing and perform when and wherever possible. My family was theater people. My sister Dorothy was singing in a musical in London and I was ready to try my hand as well. At my first audition for a London musical, I was told, "Don't call us, we'll call you." However, after my next audition I was finally in show business. My theatrical career was off to its start and I went from show to show, learning all the time. I was often told that I had a wonderful tenor voice and should be making records. Like all aspiring actors, I wished to further my career, so I set about getting more artistic exposure. In a music publisher's office one day while singing through Mario Lanza's song "Because You Are Mine,' a producer from MGM records heard me and asked me to audition. Two days later I was at Abbey Road, the famous recording studios in London, auditioning. Two weeks later, at the same facility with a forty-piece orchestra, I made my first professional recording, an exciting event comparable perhaps to finishing one's first marathon. The record was moderately successful but after several weeks of airtime throughout England and selling thirty thousand copies, it was dropped.

I continued practicing my singing and auditioning and also took a job in a big London department store at night so I could provide for my growing family of three boys. It was a frustrating time artistically, so after months of deliberation I decided to go to Canada and stay with relatives while exploring my options there. While on passage to Canada aboard ship, I practiced my singing in the ship's theater when no one was there. A couple heard me and loved my singing. They knew an agent in Chicago and encouraged me to audition, but of course I couldn't just get up and go to Chicago, as I had to earn a living. They eventually sent me a hundred dollars to get to Chicago and audition, and the agent landed me a job singing with an international ice show. For nine months I worked two shows every night. I did not realize it at the time, but my vocal training, which involves lots of deep breathing and chest expansion, would have an impact on my running career thirty years later.

After the ice show I put together my own nightclub act and

toured the United States playing in mostly respectable, but sometimes dumpy, nightclubs. I made a living, enough to support myself and my family back in England, but it was a far cry from what I had hoped. My marriage didn't last and I missed my boys, but felt driven to achieve some kind of success in my chosen profession before I could return to England. It is an unfortunate fact that the vast majority of trained and capable actors and singers are unemployed most of the time.

Through sheer cussedness (a personal quality that has helped me in my world-record running attempts) I stuck with my plan, enjoying a long and gratifying theatrical career which I continue to do today though on my own terms and when it doesn't interfere with my running.

After trying my hand in Hollywood with no success, I took a position with the prestigious Indiana University Professional Opera School to sing leading tenor roles as well as become a part-time teaching assistant. With second wife Anne and baby daughter, I moved to Bloomington Indiana. Anne got a job teaching at a local high school, and I continued to supplement my income singing every Sunday in a large church, which paid a generous stipend. It was a stressful life filled with fourteen-hour days of studying, teaching, and rehearsing. To relieve the stress, I began an exercise program, swimming one mile every day, five days a week, further developing my lungs and cardiovascular fitness.

After two years of this intensive life at the university, I received a letter from my father in England. He and my mother begged me to come back for a visit. Of course I desperately wanted to, but the cost had always been prohibitive. Transatlantic air travel was not accessible to the ordinary traveler back in 1961, but after making inquiries we found a reasonable boat fare and packed up to spend the summer in England.

Seeing my parents and renewing my relationship with my three boys was just wonderful. I did a bit of auditioning while back home and started to receive positive reviews, which brought more roles. That summer in London lasted eleven years. I had reestablished my acting and singing career, working with famous stars such as Juliet Prowse, Maggie Smith and Michael Crawford. I was making a name for myself and was known as the King of TV Commercials as I had five commercials airing at the same time. A Birdseye chicken dinner ad I starred in won the Cannes Film Festival award in 1977 as top black-and-white advertisement of the year.

Acting is hard work, very physical and demanding on the body. I always stayed in somewhat good shape because I never knew what sort of part I'd be playing. At six feet tall, my usual weight is 148, and I rarely fluctuated. I grew up on the usual English diet, fish-and-chips and bangers, which isn't all that healthy but Mom lived till ninety and my Dad died at ninety-five. And of course, growing up pre–World War II, everyone walked everywhere. And those famous English gardens were maintained with loving but very physical care. We used push mowers, tilled the soil with forks and spades, worked on our hands and knees to cultivate a victory garden. It was all done manually and it was all very grueling. And like most kids, I smoked. Everyone smoked. Even my mother-in-law who owned a health food store smoked. But I got smart and quit before it ruined my voice.

After more than eleven years in England I joined the Royal Shakespeare Company on a tour that brought me back to America, to illustrious places such as the Kennedy Center and Broadway. While I was on tour an old friend called upon me and asked if I would be interested in accepting the position of Artist in Residence at Bemidji State University in Minn-esota. I was fifty years old by now and this presented an opportunity to settle down with my family, Anne and three children, so we decided to move to the Icebox of America.

The position was everything I hoped it would be. I was very involved with my students: coaching, directing, or putting on productions. A group of my students were runners and every once in a while I'd join them. After a few months of these runs they talked me into doing a 10K. I thought, Why not? I was fifty-five at the time and won my age division with a time of 44:44. After that I was hooked. I kept on racing and winning my age division, but there wasn't much competition. Never having raced before, I didn't know if I was fast or just in a slow group. Five years after my first road race I ran my first marathon, the Twin Cities Marathon, starting in Minneapolis and finishing in St. Paul. This is known as America's most beautiful urban marathon. I was nearly sixty-one years old and completed the marathon in 3:23, placing fourth in my age division. I could have run faster but, not having any experience with marathon running, I held back. A fellow I was chatting with at mile four asked me how many marathons I had run. Telling him it was my first, he replied "You are going a bit fast for your first marathon, aren't you?" So I slowed down. The whole experience was a great thrill and I felt so well afterward I remember saying, "That was easy. I could run another one right now!"

Eight months later I ran Grandma's Marathon, also in Minnesota, and finished in 2:58, taking second place in my age division. By the time I ran my third marathon in St. Louis, I knew how to pace myself and took first place in my age division with a time of 2:53.

Eventually people were telling me that not only was I fast, but I was a gifted runner. By the time I was sixty-three, I had run nine sub-three-hour marathons and was now the top sixty-to-sixty-four-year-old runner in the nation. One of my most memorable marathons was in Los Angeles in 1987. After finishing in 2:52:38 at age sixty-two, I assumed I had won my age group, but I had a plane to catch and couldn't stick around for the results. Besides, I couldn't bear spending another minute in that city. After living among the trees and lakes and sparsely populated northern Minnesota, Los Angeles was a real culture shock. Later on I was told that the actor Dick Van Dyke had taken first. I was surprised but thought, Good for him. A few days later I learned that Dick Van Dyke had only run the last mile as part of a Hollywood relay team so in fact I did win my division. And all along I thought I had been upstaged by another actor!

Another memorable marathon was the 1997 Turin, Italy, Marathon, which I ran with my fifty-year-old son. Anthony had witnessed my 3:01:35 finish in the 1995 London Marathon, where I missed setting a new world record for my age division, seventy-to-seventy-four, by twenty-two seconds. Anthony was intrigued with the prospect of running a marathon, so we trained together sometimes on roads but mostly on muddy farm trails. Both quite fast runners, we were expecting good times in Turin. Michael, another son, came with his family to cheer us on. Halfway through the course I realized we were a bit off our 6:50-per-mile pace for a sub-3:00 finish. Anthony was still looking strong so told him to go ahead. I knew something was wrong with me but I didn't realize it was hypoglycemia until I got the dizzies and started losing my hearing. The cheers and applause of the crowds kept me going, as they recognized "The Old Man" from the prerace publicity shots. I noticed many elderly folk along the route and heard them say, "È lui," "It's him. Bravo, bravo!" It was comforting having oldies of my generation urging me on. Anthony finished in 3:02:40 and I in 3:20:01. After relaxing, dining heartily, and drinking grappa and fine Piemonte wine, I was ready to go home.

I think it is my bloody-mindedness that keeps me going. At seventy-five years of age, I am not ready to say I am old yet. We are here for such a limited time; it would be a crime not to make total use of oneself. I'm not sure runners live longer, but we certainly have a wonderful quality of life. And as our times slow down, it doesn't detract from how special our sport is. It now becomes a time to appreciate that no matter where we are or how old we get, all we have to do is put on our running shoes, head out the door, and explore. I enjoy working hard at running, singing, entertaining, and most recently building a vacation home in central Oregon. I laid fourteen hundred Mexican tiles inside and erected a stone fireplace and wall. The complete project took an entire year. Here in Oregon the family gets together to ski, run, climb, bicycle, and generally use ourselves physically as well as renewing our close ties. I'm fortunate that all my five sons and daughter Pamela are athletic; it allows for pretty dynamic gatherings of our extended family. It is a delight to train and help our grandchildren become athletes also.

In the past two years I've suffered through my first two injuries and made it through unscathed. In January 1997 I was cycling over snow-covered railroad tracks and took a spill. I landed on my hip and heard it crack. A few screws, pins, and a plate later, I was up and about on crutches. Ten days later I was doing interval training with the crutches. Ten months later I ran a 5K race in Oregon, and finished in 20:32. At seventy-three, I was the oldest runner in the race. Then in January 1999 I slipped again in the snow and broke my ankle. I was in a cast for six weeks and suffered three more months of pain and swelling. Now that I'm seventy-five, my goal is to be injury-free, do more stretching, and set more world records. I credit my intense urge to run again, and run well again, as my major healing force. Fully aware that I am not going to attain such splendid race times any more, I am still a dedicated runner, still with desires and goals. I have moderated my training regimen, and of the forty-five to fifty-five miles that I try to put in weekly, almost half is walking.

Every morning I start my day with two strong cups of tea, gather myself up, get on with the day's events and somewhere fit in a run. My general philosophy is to keep moving and be kind to everyone. In 1995 I became an American citizen and I will never forget the moment at the Twin Cities Marathon in 1996 when I sang the "Star Spangled Banner" in my best operatic tenor voice. I then went to the starting line and finished the marathon in a new world record. It was my tenth try in twenty months and I finally achieved it. The featured sports story in the *Minneapolis Star-Tribune* the following day read: "A 71-year old Brit belted out the national anthem (the American one) before Sunday's Twin Cities Marathon, but it was not his high note for the day. . . . [He] waltzed to a world age-group record with a time of 3 hours, 58 seconds."

I truly think that life experiences allow us to reach a higher level, whether it's in the way we sing or run or do whatever in life brings us happiness.

ULTRA WOMAN

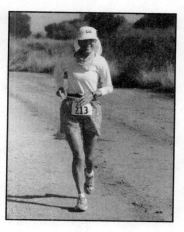

HELEN KLEIN

Date of birth: 11-27-22

Residence: Rancho Cordova, CA

"The desire of life prolongs it." —Lord Byron

Helen is in a league by herself. A retired nurse and mother of four, she took up running at fifty-five years old and hasn't stopped. From marathons to ultramarathons to the Hawaiian Ironman Triathlon to participating as a member of the American Eco-Challenge team at seventy-two, Helen believes anything is possible if it is within your grasp. One of her favorite awards is her 1995 Award for Courage in Sports. An inspiration to us all, Helen just does the best she is capable of doing and doesn't think she deserves the publicity that her dedication to exercise and fitness brings her, although she has made the experts reexamine their theories on aging and exercise.

I am an ordinary person and don't possess any special talents. I am able to do what I do mainly because of the way I was raised and in the time frame I was raised. For instance, chewing gum in school was a major offense, compared to what is allowed in schools today. My parents fostered a puritanical atmosphere where everything had to be earned, not just given. It wasn't proper to show any form of emotion, nor for women to sweat. I was raised to become a good housewife and mother and help my husband up the ladder of success, which meant staying in the background and doing a good job quietly. All of these factors have a strong impact on me today, both positive and negative. I am able to run a hundred miles because I have the desire and discipline forged from my background—but also have a hard time speaking in public or giving interviews.

In first grade I had a traumatic time learning to write because I am left-handed, something the schools didn't accept. I was forced to use my right hand and suffered through humiliations and having the pencil knocked out of my hand with a ruler until I learned to keep it in my right hand. And, taught not to display any emotion, I held it in. Till this day, I don't like to write.

For twenty years New York City was our home, where my husband and I raised our four children. I didn't work until the children were in school and then became an emergency room nurse. My career has enabled me to take care of myself and recognize problems and injuries immediately instead of putting them off, making the situation worse. After moving to Kentucky, I quit work at age fifty-three. The children were all out of the house by then and I had time on my hands. Always being blessed with good health, I wanted to continue my healthy ways, especially since I wouldn't be active at the office. Walking was my outlet, so I continued and increased my walking program just to get out and get some exercise. When I was fifty-five, Norm, my forty-year-old Type A personality husband, was challenged to a ten-mile race and recruited me to be his training partner. Neither of us had ever run before. As he conducts everything in his life, he took off with a fast start running through the streets. However, I was too embarrassed to run in shorts on the streets and be seen by everyone, so he built a track for me on our eight-acre lawn. The first few times around the track I thought I would die. But once I commit to something I don't give up so the next day I ran a little more and each day after that added one lap until I could run a mile. Within ten weeks I could run the ten miles at a twelve minute pace. I use this same formula today when I coach Team Diabetes for first-time marathoners and have a 100 percent success rate for first-time finishers. Although Norm and I finished dead last in our very first race, my only competition was from three high school girl cross-county runners so I ended up with the trophy for the masters division.

After finishing that first ten-mile race in 1978, I didn't think I could take another step. But I recover quickly and kept walking everywhere. I walk to the grocery store, take the cart home, and then bring it back. It's very efficient and I don't have to use the car as much. I decided to also continue running three miles a day for health reasons and because I had the free time. I don't go to luncheons or play bridge or things like that, so walking and running kept me busy, healthy and in shape.

In the meantime my husband decided to tackle a 26.2-mile marathon. It was always a dream he had, so fifteen months later he ran the Chicago Marathon. I had no interest at all in running with him. The ten-miler was enough for me. He tried to talk me into it, but I knew it wasn't right for me. But the marathon turned out to be a very bad experience for him, as he did everything wrong. It turned very cold in Kentucky the last few weeks of his training, so he backed off a bit. And in Chicago during that particular marathon, 1979, it turned very hot. And instead of resting the day before, taking a light meal, and getting plenty of sleep, we spent all day shopping at Eddie Bauer for clothing and equipment for our upcoming hiking trip to Nepal. Then we ate a big prime rib dinner and walked back to the hotel.

He had predicted a 3:45 finish, but by 4:00 I was getting very worried. I was waiting for him 200 yards from the finish; the plan was for me to meet him there and run with him to the finish. When I saw him, I was shocked. He looked so terrible that I was afraid for his health. His last few miles were torture. He was purple from lack of oxygen. My nursing skills immediately kicked in and soon he was breathing regularly enough to cross the finish line. I told him I would never do that again with him. I truly thought he'd be taken away in an ambulance. But he needed to run another one to redeem himself and qualify for Boston, so I knew I had to run with him to make sure he was safe. That was the beginning of my distance-running career.

Once I learned to ignore the sweat factor of distance running, I actually began to like it. And since my husband and I were going to make this a habit, I wanted to be the best that I possibly could. That goes back to the way I was brought up: Always do your best. And I also enjoyed the people we met at the races. Runners are a wonderful group of people. And there's a saying on the marathon circuit that all finishers are winners. Well, we are out there running the same course and covering the same distance as the legends such as Bill Rodgers or Frank Shorter, just a bit slower. It's quite a thrill. My goal is always just to finish; I never set a time. Actually my only goal at the finish is to look good; it helps to inspire others. It might just get a person to think about running a marathon when the person crossing the finish line looks good and feels great rather than being about to collapse. My husband is just the opposite. For him, faster is better regardless of how he looks or feels.

The next challenge my husband set for us was a fifty-mile race. And once again I took it one mile at a time, and it wasn't so bad. There was a participant in the race who was wearing an Ironman shirt; my husband took notice of that and started talking to him. Before I knew it, we were all having dinner together listening to his tales of the Hawaiian Ironman Triathlon, a three-mile swim, 112-mile bike ride, and full 26.2-mile marathon. By the time we got back to our hotel room, my husband was convinced this was his next challenge. The following day he went out and bought a bike and started to train. I told him I would run the marathon section with him, the last event of the three. He trained through the ice and snow of Kentucky but with two weeks to go he pulled his hamstring. So in February 1982 we set out for Hawaii and the Ironman competition with no idea how he would perform. He made it through the swim and the bike event but his marathon time was miserable and he vowed to come back and do a better job. After watching the Ironman as a spectator and doing the marathon part I was now convinced I could do it. Also, I suffered with him through that whole year of training and I wasn't about to do it again as a bystander. So the next day I went out and a bought a bike and started to train. I knew swimming would be my downfall, so I hired a swim coach to teach me proper form and technique. She never told me this till much later, but after our first meeting in the pool she went home and told her husband, "That woman doesn't have a snowball's chance in hell to make it." So in October of that same year, 1982, at sixty years of age I entered the second scheduled Ironman competition and finished, due to sheer perseverance.

The following year, 1983, just eight months after the Ironman, I attempted my first Western States 100 Endurance Run, which starts in Squaw Valley, California. Most people agree that between the two races, Western States is tougher and they were right. I didn't finish. I was hoping to become the first sixty-year-old woman to complete the course but had to drop out and vowed I would never again run Western States. But the next day as we flew back to Kentucky I said to Norm, "You know, if we lived in California I could train in the mountains and just maybe I could finish that thing!" Eight months later we moved to the Sacramento area and I began training, running the actual course trails every weekend. Race conditions that year were much better than the snow and ice of last year and as I finished in 29:19, I was ahead of fifteen other runners. Not bad for a sixty-one-year-old great-grandmother! Naturally I was ecstatic and knew I'd be back to do it again. And in 1986 Norm and I became the Western States race directors. I returned to the course as a participant in 1987, 1988 and 1989. 1989 was my finest year of running. At age sixty-six, I finished the Western States 100, the Vermont 100, Colorado's Leadville 100, and the Wasatch 100, in the process becoming the oldest woman to do the Grand Slam of 100-mile trail runs. I then went on to do the Angeles Crest 100, which made five 100-milers in sixteen weeks. I've learned to never say, "Never again."

I've had a great life. Norm and I are destined to do things together and we work hard at it. We started out to run the

Sahara Desert, 143 miles in six days, but Norm twisted his ankle in a water hole, probably the only one found in the desert, and had to quit. I went on to finish. There's really no limit to what a person can do, as long as there are no major health problems to hinder them. Before I tackle something I have to believe in my heart and mind that there is a possibility of finishing; then I give it my best. I have been blessed with good genes and biomechanics, but they carry you only so far. People tend to blame their ancestors for a lack of good genes, but sports doctors agree that the gene pool, whether good or not, contributes only 20 percent to performance. I can give my good genes some credit for having never been injured, but I also run relaxed; my muscles are always supple. You can also trash those good genes if you overdo it.

In 1995 I received an Award for Courage in Sports. That says a lot about how I view my challenges. Because of my age and what I do in sports, the press is everywhere I go. This makes me uncomfortable, as, going back to the way I was raised, I was taught to keep a low profile. It's difficult for me to give inspirational talks, but I do it because I believe in the message. This past October I was invited back for the Courage in Sports ceremony to give a talk. Among the people receiving the award was a young man who lost his foot in an auto accident but climbed Mount Everest with an artificial foot. Another award recipient was a single mother of four children who lost her daughter in the Columbine High School shootings. She was also recovering from surgery to remove a cancerous brain tumor. A soccer coach, she was receiving the Coach of the Year Award. In her acceptance speech she noted that she was taking the year off to raise funds to build a new school library. These people, and others like them, are inspiring, real-life proof that there is no limit to what people can do. That was the topic of my talk. It's always the topic of my talks.

My husband, children, grandchildren, and great-grand-children are all very proud of my accomplishments. When I completed the last leg of the 100 Grand Slam, they hung a huge banner at the finish line that said, GRAND SLAM CONGRATS TO GRANDMA RUNNER. They each have their hand-prints painted on with little notes. It now hangs in my office. I already have big plans for 2000. I would like to run the Leadville 100 this year and give it one more shot now that I'm seventy-seven. I'm also currently training for my next fifty-miler in March. Then I have my team coaching, which takes up weekends for the actual training and at least one night a week for lectures. Then there are my race director-ships and my daily exercise. I go to the gym three times a week for weight training and I do yoga every morning and get in my daily four miles. "Work hard and keep busy" is another motto of mine.

I've done incredible things in my life but I don't think it warrants the attention I receive. I know there are millions of people out there who can do what I do but are unaware of it. A third grader once said to me, "I don't know anyone like you. Most of the seventy-year olds I know lie on the couch all day and complain about their aching backs."

Walter Bortz, author of *We Live Too Short and Die Too Long*, is a good friend of mine. When he gave me a copy of that book he told me I would most likely live to 125. Now he has another book called *Dare to Be 100*, and I kid him that he just deducted 25 years from my life span!

THE JUMPING-JACK MAN

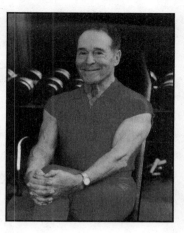

Jack LaLanne

Date of birth: 9-26-14

Residence: San Luis Obispo, CA

"People don't die of old age, they die of inactivity."
—Jack LaLanne

Is there a person in America over the age of fifty who hasn't heard of Jack LaLanne? Often called The Godfather of Fitness, Jack is in as much demand today at eighty-six as he was during his television show days back in the 1950s. As a sought-after public speaker, his audiences include his longtime supporters and a new group, college kids. Jack has dedicated his entire life to proper diet, fitness, and good mental health, and his methods are scientifically sound. What he preached from the beginning, and was sometimes criticized for, is now gospel to millions of Americans who want to get in shape and stay in shape. Besides having a wonderful sense of humor, Jack is as strong as ever and still producing books and exercise tapes along with his wife, Elaine. The man who said, "Better to wear out than rust out," is still on top of the world.

My memories of growing up are not pleasant. I was a mean, irritable, forty-pound-underweight, skinny troublemaker with pimples and boils. When the boys weren't beating me up, the girls were. My life was sheer hell. Without realizing it, I had become addicted to the sugar my mother gave me as a constant treat. The more I misbehaved, the more sugar she gave me to appease my nasty nature. It was a vicious cycle. By age fifteen I suffered from blinding headaches and suicidal mood swings. Even took a knife to my brother. The processed sugars inside me had created a monster.

Desperate for help, my mother dragged me to hear a pioneer nutritionist, Paul Bragg, speak at the Oakland City Women's Club. After hearing him speak I realized I was addicted to sugar. Bragg took me under his wing and promised that if I exercised and ate a proper diet, I could achieve good health. Well, I believed him and started out the very next day to build a new Jack LaLanne. Besides, I wanted to date girls and become an athlete, and if this was going to get me there I was all for it. The first thing I did was pray to God to help me cut out the sugar. The next thing I did was join the Berkeley YMCA, where two guys kept weights locked up in a box. They let me use them after I wrestled them down on a dare. Along the way I became a vegetarian and swore off white flour and white sugar. My motto became, "If man makes it, don't eat it."

The positive changes occurred immediately. My temperament changed and I became a different, more settled kid in the house. Everyone noticed the new me. I became a voracious reader and absorbed everything that would help me improve myself. I wanted muscles, lots of them. *Grey's Anatomy* became my bible; I wanted to know how the body performs. Like a born-again bodybuilder, I went crazy and built a gymnasium in my backyard with all sorts of crudely made equipment such as makeshift weights, climbing ropes, chinning bars, push-up and sit-up machines. This was 1931 and I was seventeen years old. As word got out, firemen and policemen started coming around to see what the neighborhood kid had put together. Not many people had heard of bodybuilding before and here I was, not only doing it and showing off the results but also teaching the program to the firemen and policemen. They all became LaLanne converts and before I knew it, I had my first gym. I finally decided to charge five dollars a month to train people.

During college I studied premed and also went to chiropractic college and graduated with a degree in chiropractic medicine. Wanting to share my enthusiasm and knowledge with others, I decided to open the nation's very first modern health studio in 1936 on the third floor of an old office building in downtown Oakland, California, paying forty-five dollars a month in rent. I was twenty-one years old with just enough money to get going. No one was beating down my door at first. In fact, the only exercise I got was looking out the window and watching all the people pass by. The local high school coaches refused to let their players come. Told them weight lifting would make them muscle-bound. Even the doctors told their patients to stay away from me. Told them lifting weights would lead to heart attacks and they would lose their sex drive and men wouldn't get erections. One of my members, about my only member, was Trader Vic of the restaurant business. He stopped by early in the morning for a massage. He believed in me and wanted to help and gave me the best advice I ever received. He said, "Jack, if the people don't come to you, you have to go to them." That got me into action. I went to Oakland High School and started lecturing the kids on exercise and fitness. They all knew me as a fitness guru but weren't about to give up their sweets and sodas. So I picked out the fattest kid and the skinniest kid and went to their homes and spoke with their parents. This was very hard for me, because I was a very shy person. I'd walk around the block to get up the courage, ring the bell, and hope nobody was home so I could leave. But I believed in myself and that gave me the courage and determination to keep going and give the parents my prepared spiel. I told them I would take fifteen pounds off the fat kid and get his waist down three inches in thirty days or I would double their money back. I told the skinny kid's parents I'd put fifteen pounds of solid muscle on him and add two inches on his arms, three inches on his chest and double his strength in thirty days or I would double their money back. I did this fifty times and had fifty successes. One boy lost 111 pounds in eight months. These kids became my kids. I taught them to dress properly, told them how important school was. In fact, if their grades fell below a C, I'd kick them out. I became their confidant, instructor, and friend because I always told them the truth. Within a year I had to shut down the membership because I was so busy. I went from being a charlatan to having the dads come and ask if I could squeeze them in. But they didn't want anyone to know they were working out so I had to open the gym early in the morning or after hours and keep it secret. Then the ladies started coming and wanted it kept a secret. I was the first one to have women work out with weights. Before long it started to look like a psychiatrist's office, with secret doors so no one could see who was coming or going. Then I had to build a separate space for the ladies because nothing was co-ed back then. Soon afterward a health food store was added, and then a restaurant.

In 1951 I was approached to do a television show in San Francisco that broadcast to the Bay Area each morning. The show started out with a motivational talk about how it's never too late to start and the belief that anything in life is possible if you make it happen. Then we moved on to nutritional tips and then exercises viewers could do in their own homes. The chair became very famous. In fact, one viewer wrote in, "Jack, I've been watching your show for ten years and that chair hasn't lost a pound." Well, the rest is history. My show aired for more than thirty years. Yami yogurt was one of my first sponsors, then I sponsored myself with products I believed in. When the show moved to Hollywood in 1953 it was picked up by more than two hundred affiliate stations and seen nationwide. Housewives were my target; I loved to tease them with my classic one-liners such as, "Ten seconds on the lips, a lifetime on the hips," and, "Your waistline is your lifeline."

The best part of getting my TV show was meeting my future wife, Elaine. She was working a show from four-thirty to six, and the first time I saw her she was munching on a chocolate doughnut. My first words to her were, "You know, the only thing good about that doughnut is the hole in the middle." She laughed and kept munching away. We've been married now for almost fifty years and have three children. We've made a great team all these years and the reason for our success, both professional and personal, is that "she's always right!" She is the power beneath my muscle.

I continued to live the life I believed in and made every day count toward a positive lifestyle in my diet and fitness routine. My message has survived through the years because I speak the truth and I am always willing to show the world that "I put my muscle where my mouth is." Turning forty, I swam the length of the San Francisco Golden Gate Bridge underwater with 140 pounds of equipment, including two air tanks, an undisputed world record. Turning sixty, I swam from Alcatraz Island to Fisherman's Wharf, handcuffed, shackled and towing a thousand-pound boat. My seventieth birthday was spent handcuffed with my feet shackled towing seventy boats with seventy people from the Queen's Way Bridge in Long Beach Harbor, California, to the Queen Mary, one and a half miles. And I've already planned my next feat when I turneighty-seven. I am going to swim twenty-six miles underwater from Catalina Island to Los Angeles. That is, if Elaine doesn't divorce me, as she has promised she will if I do any more of these feats.

I do these incredible feats to bring attention to my profession. People need role models. They need to see an eighty-year old man doing things unheard of, but I can do them because I've practiced my own preaching all these years. My top priority in life is my workout every day. Sure it's hard to get out of a hot bed next to a hot woman at four-thirty in the morning. I hate it but I do it. I just don't listen to that little devil standing on my shoulder telling me to stay in bed. My routine is the same as it's always been: Get to the gym by five-thirty and do one hour of heavy weight training followed by one hour of water exercises done aerobically, which I call my hydro-nastics workout. I change my program every three to four weeks. Once your body gets accustomed to a particular program, it stops responding.

The body is an amazing machine, and we have to learn to take care of it. There are 640 muscles in the human body, and I take every one into account as I plan and demonstrate an

exercise routine. The human body is fearfully and wonder-
fully made, and regular exercise will cleanse it of most ingest-
ed pollutants. This is a God-given machine and the only way
you hurt it is not to use it. They've done experiments with
ninety-five-year-olds and doubled their strength, vitality and
energy in eight weeks. You can reverse the aging process.
Give me a seventy-year-old who has never exercised a day and
I'll give you back a stronger person. It doesn't make any difference if the person is five or seventy-five; they can both do
something to better themselves. Imagine you're at the bottom
of the Empire State Building in New York and want to get to
the top and the elevator is out. An athlete will get up the
fastest. An old man will get up too, but much slower, taking it
a step at a time. It's the same thing in working out. It takes
time and you have to know how to pace yourself. Make haste
slowly and you'll see the results. What the mind can conceive,
the body will achieve.

I've been in this business so long, I don't ever have to BS
anyone about anything. Sometimes I'm asked how I feel now
about all the criticism I endured back when I was starting
and I say what Jesus said on the cross: "Forgive them, for
they knew not what they did." It is most gratifying to see that
everything I have preached for seventy years, not only regarding exercise but nutrition as well, is coming to fruition.
Yesterday I was a crackpot and today I am an authority. My
biggest fans now are the young people, from college kids to
baby boomers, along with my loyal followers. I have no
patience with people who sit on the couch and blame God or
somebody else for their failings. Well, God helps them who
help themselves. Older people don't feel old unless they are
told they're old. I know people who died at forty and were

buried at seventy. Everything in life that is meaningful, everything from working out to sex, takes time and energy. People
get lazy. Find a hobby, start a business, do something, anything
to get off your butt. I worked hard to get where I am today.
Heck, I'd be six-foot-five if I wasn't beaten down so much.

There is still so much I have to get done. I'm coming out
with a new videotape and I am planning to make one especially for people who are wheelchair-bound or bedridden.
They can still exercise—it just takes the know how. If you
have an injury or a weak spot you can still work around it;
other parts of the body will adapt. Elaine and I travel
throughout the world lecturing and inspiring people to reach
greater heights through exercise and nutrition. Women come
up to me and tell me how they worked out with me on TV
back in the 1950s and that they still have their Glamour-
stretchers. Many of today's exercise gimmicks are misleading.
You can't tell someone they are going to be a different person
in three minutes a day. If you do nothing but use a butt-mas-
ter and don't eat properly, your butt will get bigger! Everyone
wants a quick fix but it doesn't work that way.

I know I am going to make a hundred. Believe me, I can't
die. It would ruin my image.

LIFE AT EIGHTY IS FULL OF PANACHE AND VIGOR

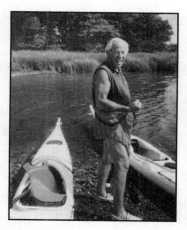

LEONARD LESHAY

Date of birth: 5-5-19

Residence: Fresh Meadows, Queens, New York

"Grow old along with me! The best is yet to be, the last of life for which the first was made." —Robert Browning

Lenny knows the secret to aging. He doesn't admit to this, but it's his humor. That and his kayaking. It's something he loves and does all the time, even through the winter. It's what makes him happiest— his boat and the ocean. Kayaking combines a sense of mental and physical exercise that relaxes him and clears his head. He paddles all over the East Coast but is especially fond of the waters around his home in Fresh Meadows. He's led a good clean life, still works in the garment center in New York City and is always on the look-out for a girlfriend. At eighty, Lenny may be the oldest paddler on the water, but he is also the youngest at heart.

You want to know the secret to growing old gracefully? It's real simple. Stay away from old people. That, and younger women will keep you young forever. I spent my eightieth birthday this year kayaking with friends, including quite a number of young women, in the waters around my neighborhood. I've paddled all over the East Coast, but this area, Three Village waters, is particularly beautiful. I couldn't imagine spending my birthday any other way.

I was born in my house on Mohegan Avenue and the delivery fee was two dollars. The Bronx back then was the garden spot of New York, all woods. My buddies and I would ride our bikes over to Yonkers and go fishing and hunting. By fourteen we were camping out all night in the woods around my house. We were always active, never bored. There were a million things to do after school, starting with my paper route and then finding my friends to go hiking through the woods. As Christians, their favorite song was "Onward Christian soldiers, and don't forget Lenny." We built some amazing tree forts. I didn't enjoy competitive sports, thought chasing after balls seemed silly. I was always a water rat, though. Bought my first boat at eighteen, a wooden canoe for fifteen dollars. Rigged a sheet to it and sailed off the shore of City Island in the Bronx. My friends called it the *Plastic Wood* because it was patched so many times.

After the Bronx, my family moved to an apartment and kept moving all over the city. My mother hated to have the place painted, so instead of painting we moved. Graduating from DeWitt Clinton High School in 1937, which was all boys then, I went to work in the garment district, where my dad was a salesman. My father made a comfortable living, but worked too hard at achieving it. Everybody in the garment district knew Ben LeShay; they called him the Mayor of Seventh Avenue. Great-looking man. He died at seventy-six from a heart attack while commuting home on the Long Island Rail Road. It was the stress that did him in.

For four years I worked on Seventh Avenue and discovered girls. That's when life got exciting. But my career was short-lived, as the army came calling. For the next three and a half years I lay telephone lines for the troops. While I was away, I dreamed of concrete sidewalks, milkshakes, and women. The best part of the war was the year I spent on Bora Bora where the native population was 1,200, which included 150 single women to 149 enlisted army men. We had a great time together.

In 1945 I returned home from the army and spent all my savings. Bought a car, traveled, dated, and finally went back to work in the garment district. Been there ever since and never intend to retire. One of the secrets to living life successfully is being a part of something, being connected. I want to be connected to my work, my family, my girlfriends, and the water forever. So far I'm doing a good job at it.

One of the best things that ever happened to me was getting married. Even though she couldn't swim and didn't like boats, I was willing to give all that up for her. For thirty years we had a good, happy marriage. Then my wife developed a brain tumor. After the operation the doctors said, "Mr. LeShay, we have good news and bad. The good news is that we removed the tumor. The bad news is that it's too late." Nine months later she died in my arms.

After she passed away I discovered the water and boats again and bought myself a canoe. Took that thing everywhere, going out around Stony Brook, up the Connecticut River and Saranac Lake. When I was sixty-two I started dating a young woman, a nurse who was thirty-nine; just the perfect age. We really hit it off and became good friends. In fact, we became such good friends over the years that we decided to get married. We spent the weekends in the canoe following the waterways. Both longtime smokers, we decided to give it up. From four packs a day for forty years I went cold turkey. To tell the truth, I was thinking of quitting. Got tired of burning holes in my suits and standing in a pile of butts at the end of the day. In two weeks, we were over the habit. Unfortunately she died of a heart attack before we were married.

I was back on the water again, alone. It's where I go for solitude and mental housecleaning. The canoe was getting difficult to handle solo, so the following year I attended the boat show looking for something different. I noticed these kayaks, which were easy for one person to handle and navigate. At sixty-eight years old I discovered a new love in kayaking. I also discovered a new girlfriend who liked to kayak. Life was good again. I'm attracted to the younger women because they are active and fun to be with. Sometimes the older ones, they kvetch too much. I keep a spare kayak for the girlfriends. It makes a great opening line. And if they don't like the water or kayaks, they're history. I dump them right away.

For the first few years, I was the only kayaker out there. It was peaceful, but lonely. Joining the Metropolitan Association of Sea Kayakers was a great opportunity to meet fellow water lovers. Although the average age in the club is forty-five, I more than keep up. I can never get enough of kayaking. It's the thing that makes me happiest. That and still working every day in the garment district. Never took a sick day, I'm not on any medication, don't even feel an occasional pang of arthritis, and everything still works.

Kayaks are the best way to see and appreciate the waterways around here. There is some stunning natural beauty you can only get to see on a kayak: horseshoe crabs, swans, egrets, cranes, the marshes are my favorite spots. You can always catch something mating. The nicest part of kayaking is that it is a twelve-month sport. You don't ever have to come in off the water.

However, there was one time the water almost did me in. A few buddies and I decided to go out on a February weekend. They were the best of the paddlers. As we headed out the Connecticut River, the gusts were picking up and the water got really choppy. My boat tipped and I couldn't right myself, thought I was going to drown. My buddies pulled me up, righted the kayak, and dragged me and boat to shore. The cold wind was cutting through me, and they knew it was only a matter of time before the symptoms of severe hypothermia took hold. They dragged me to the nearest house and knocked on the door for help. Turns out it was a convent, and the nuns graciously took me in and cared for me. Not bad service for a good Jewish boy.

During the weekends I'm up at 5 A.M. and on the water by 10. The entire day is spent gliding peacefully by—not racing, just cruising. If you go too fast, you're bound to miss something. It clears my head. There's no stress. I won't have to worry about having a heart attack on the train like my dad. This is just more than just physical exercise for me. It's a mental exercise that keeps me young at heart, surrounded by young-at-heart people. They're half my age but they treat me like an equal. Once you start thinking you're old, you might as well think you're dead. I have a buddy I've known since we were twelve years old. He calls me every once in a while, but he is a pain in the neck to talk with. All he does is complain: This hurts, that aches, I'm taking this medication, I feel half dead. His phone call is nothing but a list of complaints and ailments. I love the guy, but I don't want to hear that stuff.

A few times a year our group paddles around the island of Manhattan, a thirty-three-mile trip that takes us about eleven hours. Shoving off at Liberty State Park in New Jersey, we paddle past the Statute of Liberty, up the East River, and cross over to the Jersey side. Breaking for lunch, we pull up at a beach along the Palisades and then cruise the Hudson back home. It's very strenuous but a fun trip, well worth it. You have to be in shape to do this sort of thing because when twenty-mile-an-hour wind gusts come up and the tide is against you, well, let's just say it's one hell of a workout. The last trip we made was this past August, a few months after I turned eighty. No one has the nerve to call me "Pop." If they did, I'd kill them.

You know, I've been lucky. Good clean living, no complaints, and plenty of girlfriends. I watch very little TV, maybe a few old *Star Trek* episodes. I baby-sit my two-year old grandson but make it clear I don't change diapers. Never did. Don't go to the gym, eat anything I want, and enjoy every day. I don't baby myself or complain. If I catch a cold, I don't angst. It will go away. Why bother worrying? No one gets off this earth alive anyway. I don't ever plan on retiring; in fact I still get job offers. Couldn't retire if I wanted to.

You want to know my secret? Have a good life. And right now, mine couldn't be better. For my eightieth birthday I got a new kayak, and a new car. Now all I need is a new girlfriend to share them with.

BIKER CHICK

LOIS LINDSAY

Date of birth: 1-1-35

Residence: Boise, Idaho

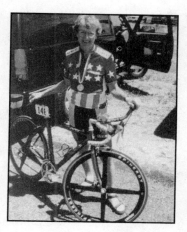

> "Cycling provides all the great lessons in life:
> humility, pride, greed, discipline, grappling with the ego,
> and learning what your will is and when to apply it."
> —**John Weissenrider**

When I spoke with Lois for the first time, I realized she was a perfect fit for the book. Dedicated to raising her children and following her husband from base to base while in the air force during the Vietnam era, Lois finally took on something just for herself at the age of forty-two, when she hopped on a bicycle. It transformed her life and she became a major competitor in the mostly male-dominated world of bike racing. Through the exercise and fitness routine she follows to stay so fit, she has earned four national cycling titles. Lois also looks and feels years younger than her age. At sixty-five years old she is speeding up, not slowing down.

Growing up on a farm taught me discipline and structure at an early age, but it also taught me I didn't want that life. My parents were tired all the time. The tasks are a never-ending cycle of rising early, feeding the animals, doing all the chores, getting to bed late, and starting the cycle over again. It was a real struggle and we were poor, but there was always food on the table. However, we didn't have any savings or extra spending money.

In school my goal was to become an artist. You can't get much farther from farm life than that. My notebooks were covered in doodles and sketches. There were no sports to talk about; I didn't even own a bike. I remember some track meets in grade school, but that's it. In high school gym class we did the bare necessities, some softball, basketball on half courts, just moving around. After high school I attended the University of Idaho to study art. There, I met my future husband, who also grew up struggling on a farm in Wilder, Idaho. He was studying agricultural education with the hopes of becoming a teacher. But what he dreamed about was becoming an air force pilot. His dream came true, and we got married after he was commissioned a second lieutenant from college. I dropped out my junior year to be able to travel with him on his stations of pilot training. During his twenty-five-year career we had three children and eighteen different addresses. Our longest and most memorable station was living in Japan. This was in the early 1960s when Vietnam was getting to be a political hot seat. He was assigned a tour over there while we stayed in Japan and then the Philippines. It was a very depressing time for us. Many of our friends were killed and a quarter of his squadron was lost. We lived on the edge of emotional stress. After his tour was up we were transferred to Florida, but he signed up for several one-year tours and went back to Vietnam. He just loved flying. During this time I also got my pilot license at Clark Air Force Base in the Philippines and also illustrated a book about our experiences in

Japan and the Philippines.

When he finally settled down for a reasonable amount of time, the kids were in high school and we lived in Virginia. This was now the mid-1970s. My husband had already taken up biking as a way to stay fit when he wasn't flying. He commuted on his bike to the airfield and back. With only one car, which I was in most of the time shuffling the kids around, biking became his alternative mode of transportation. Even took a few courses in how to fix and build his own bike. In Virginia my son also got interested in biking, so they joined a club together and started going to a few local races. I was forty-two at the time and went to their races to cheer them on. After a few races I thought, "I can do this!" Up to this point I was a stay-at-home mom, basically an almost single parent when my husband was away on his tours of duty. My life consisted of driving the kids everywhere, doing all the volunteer jobs at school, church, and in the communities where we lived, but I had never done anything just for myself. Bike racing looked exciting and I did see a few women on the course, which gave me some confidence that just maybe I could do it.

The next day I went out and borrowed a small, woman's-style bike from a friend and rode seven miles. Not being in shape, I was totally exhausted. Actually, I was wasted! Thoughts like, Why did I do this? crept through my mind. I had no endurance. When I tried to ride with my husband and son, I couldn't keep up with them. Biking is hard work. But something was calling me. Despite the pain and tiredness, it was exhilarating. What I needed was a training routine and started slowly building up, going a little farther each day. But as I conquered one obstacle, whether it was a hill or a sharp turn or learning to control the speed, there was always another one looming in the distance. Every incline looked like Mount Everest. However, instead of giving up I started to concentrate on my achievements—on how far I'd come since that morning I rode seven miles—and I'd be encouraged to face the next obstacle. I now knew I could conquer whatever came my way. Along with the training, I began running a mile each day to build my endurance; soon I could go out for longer distances at greater speeds. My goal was to be able to ride comfortably with my son and husband and I was there, had reached my first of many goals. Eventually I worked my way up to completing a century, one hundred miles. It took over eight hours to complete. It was very strenuous and I worked particularly hard on that ride, as I didn't want to embarrass myself in front of the other riders.

The century ride whetted my appetite for more. I wanted to work even harder and improve. I was hooked, got totally caught up with my biking career. The kids and my husband were very supportive. One thing I learned about myself through biking was that I had a very competitive spirit. I wanted more, wanted to start racing, wanted to start winning at racing. When I'd be out on a ride with other people little thoughts crept into my head, such as, I bet I could beat that person, I bet I could go faster and pass them. Three years after first hopping on my neighbor's bike, I entered my first competition. My husband had already been racing with the U.S. Cycling Federation, which sponsors annual national championships. Every time he'd come home from the nationals he would encourage me to participate. Bikers from all over the country compete. He knew I'd love it and would fit in perfectly. To enter the nationals, you have to be a licensed rider and qualify in the required time trials, so this was a big deal. I trained very, very hard. The trials were in Hawaii, where we were living at the time, but the course was very hilly, very difficult. I finally made it to the nationals, which were being held in Milwaukee, Wisconsin, in 1979 at the age of forty-four. I was so nervous; I couldn't sleep the night before and arrived at the starting line totally fatigued. Then I made a decision to pace myself with the fastest riders. Big mistake. Maintaining speeds of twenty miles per hour was nerve-racking and I worried about falling. These women were experienced racers and I was just a scared novice. The course was twenty-five miles and I placed tenth in my age group. I was discouraged but glad for the opportunity to finally be a part of the big arena. I was totally intimidated by the other women who were the best in the country. It was a very humbling experience for me, a beginner.

The only way to get better at racing was to enter more races, so I did just about every local race that came up. But I had a major setback in my training in 1980, while preparing for the National Championship to be held in Bisbee, Arizona. I was visiting my sister at her farm and decided to take my bike out to do some speed training on the backcountry roads surrounding the farm. At the height of my speed, I saw a dog out of the corner of my eye but didn't think he'd be stupid enough to come after me, as I was flying. Well, he was that stupid and ran right into my frame. I went down hard. I hate to admit this but I wasn't wearing a helmet at the time and the first thing I noticed was all the blood dripping down into my face. It was a bad crash. I could barely pull the bike off my body with all the pain and wasn't able to move my arm. Thirteen stitches and a dislocated shoulder later, I learned never to ride without a helmet again. By the way, the dog was fine. After that episode I never go out without a can of pepper spray to deter the next dog that wants a bite out of my bike.

My only bike was totaled. I couldn't afford a new one, so my husband rebuilt the broken one for me. Between my injuries and fixing the bike, I was looking at three months out of training, so it was back to running. This time I decided to do some interval speed work while running. The idea of running a marathon began circling through my head. I met another runner who had completed over a dozen marathons and she offered to train me. In retrospect, giving only three months to train for a marathon wasn't a very smart idea but at the time I needed a goal to get through the three months. A setback like I experienced, my injuries and losing my bike, was devastating. It's not only physical pains but emotional as well. To get through the emotional pain, I ran like a maniac. The training was very hard, very different from biking. When you get a blister from running, you can't run. But you can bike with blisters. After the three months I was ready to run the 1980 Honolulu Marathon. Biking and running are somewhat complementary, but not when it comes to extreme distances like a marathon versus a century. Different parts of the body are being used and, if not conditioned, begin to rebel. During the 26.2 miles, those blisters came back to haunt me, and I often took walk breaks. My back also decided to start complaining, something I never experienced in biking. My only goal was to finish, not to run for a time, and it paid off. I accomplished my goal, but I couldn't wait to get back on the bike.

Finally back to biking, I started training with my husband and the experienced club riders who taught me about pacing, drafting, climbing—all the things I didn't know that would make me a better racer. The hard work and effort paid off and by the time I entered my fourth nationals in 1986 I set a record in my age group at the 40K time trial. I was overcome with emotion. It was a wonderful lesson that all the grueling work was worth it. For every doubt I ever had, for every fall, for every sore muscle, winning was the culmination.

Turning fifty-eight in 1993, I was invited to join a masters cycling team to Russia. It was a goodwill trip to promote camaraderie through biking. I was thrilled to be asked and found myself in a small town in Russia among people who had never met Americans. It was a most amazing experience, which began with a warm, cordial reception and continued for twelve days of bike racing with foreign women and making friendships. We did completely new forms of racing, like obstacle courses and sprints, which the American team had never done before. I was amazed at the life of these Russian women, who lived in poverty-like conditions on farms, got up early to milk the cows, feed the children, and then race their bikes. They were incredible! The entire town came out to support the event. They even swept the streets so we'd have a smoother course. We were treated like celebrities, and it was a lifetime thrill to be a part of it.

Last year I suffered another setback, falling down the stairs and cracking my ribs. That took three months to heal. I couldn't take deep breaths so biking was out of the question unless it was a gentle, short ride. I was sixty-four at the time and when I went to the doctor after the accident, he told me, "A woman your age shouldn't be on a bicycle." That didn't set well with me, and I told him in no uncertain terms my opinion of his advice. Six months later I competed in the nationals in St. George, Utah, so I guess that was my sweet revenge against the doctor's warning.

I do feel that women get shortchanged when it comes to biking. It's very demanding, so they initially get discouraged and if no one is bolstering them and giving much-needed support they drop the sport. Women need to believe that they can accomplish sports and it's all right to sweat, compete and be the best they can. I was never introduced to sports or given any incentive to pick up a sport throughout my life. It took me until forty-two years of age to make my own decision about picking up biking, and that was based on thinking it would be fun, something to share with the family. I never dreamed that biking, or any sport for that matter, would change my life so dramatically. Through my chosen sport I've been able to travel around the world, run a marathon as a sideline, stay in unbelievable shape, and as an added bonus eat whatever I want! Nutritionally speaking, I would say my diet was average, not the best. I still have a passion for chocolate. But biking burns off any excess fat, so I have to eat and eat well. Bikers have to learn how to eat and ride at the same time, or we "bonk," which is the biking-lingo equivalent to hitting the wall in running. I've "bonked' many times, getting dizzy and not being able to focus on the course. To avoid all that I carry nutrition bars or liquid supplements with me at all times.

Recently I picked up a new sport, Nordic skiing, as a wintertime cross-trainer. It beats having to stay indoors riding a stationary bike during the Idaho cold winds and snow. It's a tough sport, sort of a cross of skating and skiing. Not many women are doing it; I usually find myself the only female competitor my age at the races. But sometimes I get so tired and discouraged after a long workout, and have my doubts whether I can do this. The other day, I was completing my workout and came back into the lodge feeling somewhat down and depressed, mumbling something about hanging up the skis for good. A group of younger women who had recently picked up the sport overheard me and said, "Oh, you can't quit. You're our inspiration, our hero." That certainly gave a much-needed boost to my mood.

At sixty-five, I feel healthy, look healthy and know I am the best I can be. Two years ago I attended my forty-fifth high school reunion back in Weiser, Idaho. Out of the initial class size of about eighty-five, thirty-five showed up. Many of the others had already died! I looked around the room and felt that I looked much younger than the rest of the gang. I felt absolutely glowing with health. And I owe that to sports and exercise.

To sum up my life through sports, I was not born athletic, didn't have any role models in my family to follow, and could have easily turned into a couch potato like some people I know. But one of the nicest things about finding a sport regardless of age is that you can become an athlete at any stage of life. Most people don't understand how much time, energy, and dedication are needed to perform well. They give up at the early stages of exercise with excuses a mile long: "I don't like to sweat, I don't have the time, it hurts, why bother?" It's the staying power, the determination, and the dedication that make the difference between the haves and the have-nots. But once you cross the line and become a 'have', you never go back!

EXERCISE AS A LIFELONG PURSUIT

Mae MacKay

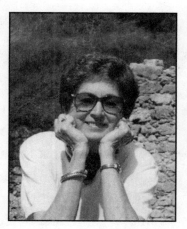

Date of birth: 5-16-21

Residence:
Palm Beach Gardens, Florida

> **"Pick the right grandparents, don't eat or drink too
> much, be circumspect in all things, and take
> a two-mile walk every morning."**
> **—Harry Truman's prescription for reaching eighty.**

Mae cared for a terminally ill husband for fifteen years. Always a vital woman who believed in living a healthy lifestyle, she was not one to complain or despair over her plight when she was widowed at sixty-five. She turned her misfortune around and created a new and exciting life, one that included bike treks across Europe, walks along the Great Wall of China, and a new boyfriend. When other women her age worried about being too careful and cautious regarding physical exercise, Mae had no such worries. Mae is now living the life she once dreamed of. Just don't tell her she is remarkable or exceptional. She thinks everyone is like her. What is probably more accurate is that every woman could be like her.

If I am going to tell you about my life, then we have to start with my mother. She was a wonderful role model. I have a picture framed in my mind of her, wearing a starched white dress with proper oxfords and her hair neatly pulled back and pinned in a bun. She was a very elegant woman. She suffered from a back condition, and although exercise was not condoned for women back then, she did "bend-overs"—as she called them—on a flat board to help strengthen her muscles. She was always ahead of her time.

Both my parents were very active and loved to travel. My father was a competitive runner, and he and his brothers were Olympic contenders. He had his own business and was always busy fixing things. When I was in my teens they bought their dream house on Long Island, right by the ocean and taught us to swim. They outlived most of their friends and left me the legacy of appreciating the benefits a healthy lifestyle.

Mother was also experimental when it came to nutrition and diet. When I started having sinus problems, she took a course on the impact of food combinations and learned how to relieve sinus headaches bynot to mixing proteins with starches or dairy. My school lunch box contained fruits and vegetables instead of the usual sandwich, and a fresh container of parsley and spinach juice. Before long my sinus problems were cured.

In 1950, at the age of twenty-eight, I married and eventually had two children. Like my mother, I always kept myself fit, but it wasn't until after my children were born that I took to exercise in a big way. Call it vanity, but I wanted to keep my figure slim and trim. In those days Bonnie Pruden, a pioneer in bringing fitness into the home, was to exercise albums what Jane Fonda was to the exercise video. Every morning after the kids were off to school, I got out my mat, put on the album, and followed the illustrations on the album jacket. There was a lot of stretching. I still do some of those techniques to this day. When we purchased a television, Jack LaLanne became my new guru and I followed him religiously; even bought his "Glamour-Stretcher," a precursor of today's elastic stretching tubes popular at the gyms. I still have it!

Then I discovered yoga and could stand on my head for long stretches of time. By now my two children were teenagers, and things were going along just fine until I was thrown one of life's nasty curves.

My husband came down with spasmodic torticollis, an affliction that causes involuntary movements of the body. As the disease worsened, he had to be bedridden. With the loss of his paycheck, I had to get a job. Kathryn and Greg were in high school, a demanding time for parents, and this entire burden landed on my shoulders. I felt like a single parent. This wasn't the 1980s when moms were part of the workforce and everything from day care centers to specialty magazines offered support. In our community in the 1950s and 60s, moms stayed at home. My daily routine changed drastically. This phase of my life lasted for more than fifteen years. When Al died, it was not a heartbreaking experience; it was a relief for him and me. I don't want that to sound bitter, but there was no cure for him. His illness had drained both of us. He wanted more out of life and never got that opportunity. I wanted more out of life and now I could start over again.

The same year my husband died, I moved to Florida. This wasn't an easy decision, as by now I had a grandchild close by. However, my sister and son were down there, and the weather was definitely an advantage. So at sixty-five years old, I entered another new phase of my life.

Wanting to continue some form of exercise, I decided to take up bicycling. The fact that I hadn't been on a bike in more than fifty years didn't bother me. My neighborhood was perfectly flat and the weather usually great, so biking seemed a reasonable exercise to pursue. My kids bought me a three-speed Schwinn bicycle for my first Christmas in Florida, and little did they know it would be the beginning of new and exciting adventures for me.

Having a bike was like being a kid again. I hopped on and was amazed how quickly it all came back. I wasn't afraid, I was thrilled. Part of my resistance to the fear of falling or worse, breaking a hip or leg, was due to the fact that I was in reasonably good shape to begin with. But also, fear is not part of my makeup. I have a healthy attitude and tend to look at the positive side of a situation instead of the negative. Fear prevents us from doing things in life that could be very rewarding. I won't let that stand in my way of living a full life.

At first I used my bike to explore the neighborhood. Every time I went out I tried to do more distance, with a goal to reach ten miles. I didn't set a time frame; whenever I got there was fine with me. A few months later I reached my goal, and it felt great.

Travel was my next big interest. My personal file of places I wanted to visit was getting larger every day and now was the time. I read about a company that sponsored bicycle trips in Europe and decided that that was for me. This wasn't an age-specific tour; I didn't want that, wasn't interested in being isolated from other age groups. I was sixty-nine years old when I signed up for this trip and at times I thought, I must be crazy. What am I doing? I won't know anyone, I'll probably be the oldest member of the group. But none of that mattered; this was a challenge I wanted to face.

Boarding my flight to France, I was filled with excitement and trepidation. The first time I met with the other group members and the tour guide was at orientation the next morning. I thought the group leader was going to have a cardiac arrest when he saw me. The tour application never asked for my age, so I guess he was a bit surprised to find a sixty-nine-year old lady in his group, when the average age of the other members was thirty-something. We were provided with the bikes, and I was somewhat nervous to make the transition from my three-speed to an eighteen-speed. Actually, I was scared to death. I asked the leader, a young girl, to stay by my side the first day or two, especially as we had to ride through street traffic the first day until we reached our more scenic route along the Dordogne River. In a day or two I had the hang of it and felt comfortable. We were putting in anywhere from twenty-five to forty miles a day.

None of the other riders were even close to my age, but that never made a difference. I don't let age become a barrier. Taking the initiative, I'd start a conversation with whoever was close by. I'm very interested in people and have always been friendly. When I was raising my two kids, I loved nothing more than for them to bring their friends over to our house so I could meet them and get to know them. We'd sit at the kitchen table and talk for hours. I was interested in their plans, their outlook on life, and always put the focus on them. After all, they'd be bored to tears hearing about my day. Some older people think that the younger people should always defer to them, thats it's owed them. I don't think anything is owed to me without earning it first.

This bike tour was the most wonderful trip I ever took. It was such a refreshing eye-opener to what other things in life I could look forward to. Of course I got sore and my muscles ached, but that's normal. Two years later I took another bike trip to Austria, riding along the Danube. Elderhostel, a company that specializes in tours for older people, sponsored the trip. But I was still one of the more senior people. We didn't do as many miles per day as on my first tour but it was a nice pace, twenty-five to thirty miles a day. This group was seasoned bicycle riders and a lot of fun. That same year I went to China. This tour group was not specifically for seniors but it was a very physical trip. At one point we had to climb eighty steps—a very steep climb—in one town alone. There were some arduous places, but it was an amazing adventure. I never thought I'd walk the Great Wall, especially at the age of seventy-six.

The following year I went to Turkey, and this year my destination is a cruise around the world. The biggest challenge here is packing for four months! My boyfriend Harold is joining me on the trip and it's been an adventure already just preparing. We share a positive attitude about life, and that goes a long way in our in relationship. When I moved to Florida, I wanted a life that included men! I joined everything I could think of—book clubs, bike clubs, hiking clubs, any chance to meet people of all ages who shared similar interests. It paid off in wonderful friendships.

Some people who are getting on in their years tend to give up, stop looking at the future. That's unfortunate, because there are so many opportunities for older people to still have a meaningful life. Age has nothing to do with it; it's an outlook on life, a state of mind, and an attitude. Unfortunately in our society, *old* is also a bad word. The younger generation seem to forget they are heading in the same direction, but you can't pedal backward on this path.

There is too much isolation of the ages in our society. We've forgotten how to relate to others and need to build better bridges between the generations. Families are not as cohesive as they use to be. Grandparents either are not around, have passed on or aren't given the opportunity to interact with young children, causing them to treat older people as strangers, a different species. However, there are many programs such as Meals on Wheels, and volunteering at retirement homes or hospitals where children and young adults can interact with older people in a positive way. For me a simple game of cards with my grandchildren can make my day. That and a bike ride. Every age has something to offer—we are all unique.

THE SILVER STREAK

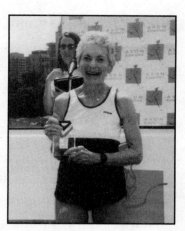

MURIEL MERL

Date of birth: 11-17-25

Residence: Pomona, New York

"The age of a woman doesn't mean a thing. The best tunes are played on the oldest fiddle." —Sigmund Z. Engel

Muriel is well known as a tough competitor at her local road races. She grew up in a multigenerational household, not leaving her parents' building until she and her husband and children bought their house in the suburbs. She feels a woman hasn't reached her prime till fifty, and then she is in for some of the best years of her life. As proof of her own philosophy, she took up running late in life and entered her first race at fifty-eight. She has never stopped, neither physically nor mentally. At seventy-four, she was the winner of her age-group prize at the New York Road Runners' annual awards night, and she manages to balance her sporting life with photography. Her physical and cerebral pursuits, along with her husband, children and grandchildren, help fulfill Muriel's life.

Born in the Bronx, I was a child of parents who came over to America from Russia and Poland. They raised me in a European manner, which meant no sports or athletic activities for girls. I never learned to roller skate, ice skate, or ride a bike. Instead the emphasis was on academics and I did very well at school, skipping grades and graduating from high school at sixteen. When I entered Hunter College, the war effort was in full swing and my then-boyfriend was drafted. I was only seventeen at the time and we thought we couldn't live without each other. Much to our parents' distress, we married. So many young couples were in the same boat and although it may seem foolish now, we did what we thought was right for us. Fortunately he survived the war, came home to me, and we've been married for fifty-seven years.

While he was away at war, I quit college and took a job. I lived with my parents and when Julius came home we continued to live with my parents, as there was a severe shortage of housing. When we were lucky enough to find an apartment, it was in the same building, which turned out to be a godsend for me as by now we were raising a family. I decided to go back to school to finish my degree. While I was at school, my parents watched the kids. It was a wonderful thing to have all three generations under one roof. My children developed a relationship with their grandparents that enriched their lives. At my mother's funeral each one of my children eulogized her with loving words and fond memories.

They say life begins at forty and that held true for me. In 1964 I received my bachelor's degree in teaching. We were finally able to buy a house, and I got my first job as a home economics teacher in the local high school. There was no time for any sports or weekday activities. But I had no complaints; life was going along at a nice pace. On weekends, my husband and I looked forward to getting out for a hike at Harriman State Park, and when our children grew older we ventured out west to hike in our national parks. The hiking kept us in good shape, but not great shape.

When I was fifty-two my husband and I planned a hiking trip to Switzerland. I knew hiking the Alps would be more strenuous than what I was used to, so I decided I needed to get stronger so I would enjoy the trip and not feel tired or worn down by the physical challenge. Running seemed the easiest and most natural way to build more endurance, and since there was a track at the school, it was also convenient. After school I'd throw on some sneakers and head over to the track. This was not a tremendous challenge but I still took it slowly, building up from a walk-run pace until I could comfortably do a steady run. The running worked and the trip to Switzerland was wonderful. This trip turned out to be a life-changing event for me. With the kids grown up and out of the house, we had time on our hands and started to hike all over the world, including trekking in Nepal. We went with adventure travel groups and were always the oldest members of the group, as we now were pushing sixty. The first time the groups came together was always the same experience for us. The other members would look at us as if to say, "Oh my God. What are they doing here?" But after the first day, we proved ourselves some of the strongest members of the group, sometimes outlasting the younger ones.

I kept up my running, plodding away on the roads and track because I saw the positive effects of what the running did for me, the benefits of staying in shape. I wasn't running races or killing myself, just maintaining my stamina. When a fellow teacher invited me to enter a local race I didn't give it much thought, but agreed to it. I am always up for a challenge, and I thought, Why not? I didn't even train for the event, which was a 7.8-mile race. That was an odd distance, but again, I didn't think much of it. The race was tiring and hard, but I placed in my age division and won a medal. Running the race was exhilarating enough, but winning something was wonderful. I had never thought of myself as competitive but something happened to me that day that I never expected to feel. I liked this running thing, especially the winning! But in reality, I probably placed in my age group because no one else my age was running.

In 1986, when I was sixty-one, a young friend asked me to enter the L'Eggs Women's 10K in Central Park with her. It seemed like a good idea, so I went. That event became a turning point for me in running. Thousands of women lined Central Park. I'd never seen anything like this in my life. By now I had been running for a few years so I knew what to expect in the race. But what I didn't expect was the number of excellent women runners. Even at my age, it was very competitive and I placed seventh in my age group. It was a big surprise to me that I could be almost as good as the top females in my division. It was very exciting. And I really pushed myself in the race to do my best. Making a vow to come back and win, two years later I placed third in my age division and in 1989 won my division, coming home with a huge silver cup. It was a revelation. At this point in my life I realized that being physically fit was a priority for me and I always made time to exercise. Other women my age would comment, "How do you fit it all in? I have no time for that." My response was always the same: "Well, that's a question of priorities. You'll make time for what matters most in your life."

I started to take my running seriously. Now I knew I was good at it and it became a passion. Retiring in 1985, I had the time to dedicate myself to serious training. Read all the books and did all the workouts. Running had changed my life and I liked the new me. I was slimmer, stronger, and felt years younger. I also ran smart so I managed to avoid any serious injuries. I was winning everything. I devoted myself to always improving. And I met some wonderful women along the way, women who were older than me and became my mentors.

We were pioneers in a sense. Not that we started the women's boom in running like Nina Kuscsik did with some of the younger women back in the 1970s, but we were pioneers for older women. We proved to everyone that it was all right, even good, for a sixty-, seventy-, or eighty-year-old woman to run. And to run well. One of my mentors was Althea Jureidini, who started running late in life and is still winning awards well into her eighties. She encouraged me to run a half marathon. Said it'd be a piece of cake for me. So I did. My son-in-law invited me to run the Philadelphia half marathon with him in 1988. I came in first in my age group. It was a wonderful experience; I even went back the next year. I was a running machine.

At sixty-five, I decided to tackle a marathon and entered the New York City Marathon. I think most serious runners always have ambitions to run a marathon, and I was no different. In fact I had been thinking about it for a while, but my husband disapproved. He discouraged me, worried that I'd get too skinny, too tired, too worn out. But this was very important to me and I knew I couldn't do it without his support. Finally, at my insistence he gave in. That marathon turned out to be my biggest challenge. The day was extremely hot and I was so worried about hydrating that I overhydrated. That can be just as bad as not drinking enough and I suffered stomach cramps, diarrhea, and nonstop bathroom stops. I did finish but it was terrible and I said, "Never again." But in spite of it all, I found myself back at the starting line two years later. This time it was much better. I trained smarter, ran smarter, and weatherwise, it was a perfect day. My whole family was there for me at points along the course. It was a great day.

Running has brought so many wonderful aspects to my life. In 1994 I was selected by Nike to be part of a commercial targeted at older athletes. The voice-over proclaimed, "I may be wrinkled and gray, but I'm not old." The thirty-second spot showed me running and lifting weights, along with other older athletes doing their sports. Even though I was sixty-nine at the time, I was the baby of the commercial. There was a seventy-six-year-old female gymnast and another seventy-one-year-old male runner from my club. It was my fifteen minutes of fame. It was very flattering but I remember how long it took them to film a thirty-second spot. Forever! Another voice-over line from the commercial was, "I don't want you to hold my hand when we cross the street unless you are my boyfriend." Nike was really trying to get the message across that older people can still excel in sports, that we should not be depicted as decrepit and incapacitated.

Another bonus from my running career was being cited in *New Woman* magazine's twenty-fifth anniversary issue in 1995. The caption read, "Uncharted territory: Aging, it's not what you think." I was seventy, an age when most women are giving up, and I was becoming famous for defying the traditional behavior of old age. This gave me pause for contemplation. What is *old*? What is *young*? Are they just words with sociological associations or can they be considered an attitude? Am I old because I can no longer hope to run a sub-eight-minute mile? I'd prefer to think I am just getting older as the natural path of life. I am still fighting not to lose my nine-minute mile. I never turn down the chance for a new experience, and I am always ready to pick up the ball and run with it. I still look forward to surprise in my life. Old? Young? Why put a handle on it? My life has been a series of turning points. Between twenty and forty, women find themselves searching for a role. For me it was raising kids, getting a degree, and teaching. The next turning point, between forty and sixty, was dedicated to working on what was in place, fine-tuning the defined roles and starting to move on and plan for the next wave. At sixty I started thinking more about myself. I wasn't ready to retire but couldn't take the unruly classrooms anymore. What would I do? Make muffins and cater? I was still young and didn't know what to do with my life. Gail Sheehy said it best in her book *New Passages:* "Find your passion and pursue it with whole heart and single mind." I have been able to do that with running and photography, my other passion, experiencing much personal gratification in these areas. I built a whole new life for myself. I don't know how I would have faced my future without them.

I am now beginning to taper off. My body isn't letting me do what I want to do anymore. Running is becoming more difficult; I'm not doing as well. I can remember when I slipped from an eight-minute mile and thinking, uh-oh. Then the 8:30 mile started to slip and I said, uh-oh again. Should I quit? I am in a new place now and don't know what to do. Do I accept the inevitable and move on? To what? I'm inching toward my next turning point, eighty and up. It's time to reflect and rethink my life, perhaps come to a compromise about my abilities and accepting my body for what it is. Whatever it brings may be difficult to internalize at first, but I will accept it. There's really no other choice. And now that I'm not able to run as fast, as long, or as hard as before, I still have my photography, which I can pursue at the same level. It's good to have both a physical and cerebral outlet.

It's been wonderful to see older women picking up sports at a late age and doing so many more things than ever before. Women are living longer and getting more and more phenomenal. When younger female friends complain about turning fifty, I tell them, "Fifty is prime! What are you whining about? This is the best time of your life." We have to work harder to do the same things men do because they are stronger. But women are proving they can hold their own. And no one better dare tell us we can't.

LIFE IS A LOT OF LUCK

JOHN MERRILL

Date of birth: 2-12-17

Residence: Waterford, CT

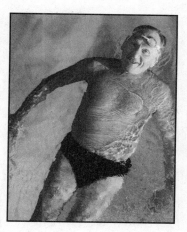

"Youth full of grace, force and fascination, do you know that Old Age may come after you with equal grace, force and fascination?" —Walt Whitman

Two words come to mind when I think of John: determined *and* busy. *The man is always up to something, whether it's writing a book about submarines or his years with the U.S. Navy Underwater Sound Laboratory, or training for his next masters swim meet. For someone who retired in 1979, his postretirement years have been extremely active. He is very computer literate, e-mailing his friends all over the country. And he loves to reminisce about growing up in depression-era Buffalo, where he just may make a visit for his high school reunion. He believes retirement gives people the chance to finally do what they want with their lives, a renewal of sorts. For John that includes swimming, writing, and being with his family. In other words, not missing a stroke.*

When I jump in the pool and put on my goggles, I don't feel eighty-two. Of course, I don't feel sixteen, either. However, the satisfaction from doing a moderate workout of about 1500 yards five times a week provides a pleasure not unlike the fun of practicing with the swim team at Lafayette High School back in 1934. I have the U.S. Masters Swimming organization to thank for my new career in competitive swimming. Before masters swimming was introduced in 1972, the opportunities for competition after high school or college were essentially nonexistent. And as a youngster growing up in Buffalo, upstate New York, the swimming environment was substantial, with natural beaches on both shores of lake Erie and the Niagara River flowing to the north along Buffalo's west border. I guess you could say swimming has always been in my blood.

In the early 1930s my friends and I would take the ferry across the Niagara River to Canada and hike to Fort Erie. Sometimes we'd fish in the river for perch. I'd sit on big bags of burlap, which lined the docks, only to discover that the bags were filled with bottles of rum waiting to be illegally transported to Buffalo at night during Prohibition. My friends and I built rafts on Frenchman's Creek and navigated around the passageways of the Niagara River, looking back across the river to industrialized Buffalo. It was a great place to grow up. Everyone comments about the amount of snow we get up there, but I can tell you I never had off for a snow day at school.

It is difficult to remember a time when I wasn't swimming. However, it wasn't till my junior year in high school that I ventured toward competition. The only requirement for being on the team was the purchase of a navy blue full-cotton suit with an L on the front. My coach concluded that my skill was in the backstroke event, although I wanted to do freestyle and long distance. Sixty-five years later and after hundreds of meets, I now realize he was right. The other activity that kept me busy during my teenage years was a paper route. They were hard to come by, as most of my peers held on to them or passed them down through the family to younger brothers or sisters. I was an only child, so I had to buy my paper route from a friend and pay him ten cents a customer. I eventually built that route up from 33 original customers to 167. And this was during the depression. My strategy was simple. I would approach customers at a busy streetcar stop and suggest they subscribe for delivery. When the depression hit hard and things got bad for my customers, I'd barter with them. I got a lot of free haircuts during that time. If people couldn't afford to pay, I didn't mind. It was the customers I knew could pay and didn't who annoyed me. I'd go back and ring their doorbell every night until they paid me.

I left high school with a desire to continue swimming but no plans as to how I'd accomplish that. I didn't realize it then, but swimming had already become an integral part of my life. Swimming also made it possible to adapt to life in unfamiliar places. Without the benefit of family or friends, swimming was my introduction to new surroundings and faces.

During the 1930s the effects of the depression were deep. There were no jobs available, so I just took more courses. I was always a good observer, always had an insatiable curiosity about how things work. In 1936 I enrolled in the New York State Merchant Marine Academy as a deck cadet. The campus was the school ship, *The Empire State*, a converted World War I freighter. In a strong hierarchy and haze-oriented environment, swimming came to my rescue. The school had a swim team and during the cadet cruise to Peru, I swam against the Bermuda Olympic Team and the Panamanian Olympic Team. My backstroke flourished during these meets and as a lowly fourth classman, I finally had an identity. Unfortunately, the academy wasn't for me, and I withdrew within the year. I didn't like the ocean; one square inch looks just like another.

Back in Buffalo, employment opportunities were still scarce. In 1938 I enlisted in the Coast Guard, which has always played a prominent role along the Great Lakes, so I grew up familiar with the Coast Guard surf stations. When I first interviewed with the guard and learned about the surf-man position, I didn't sign up right away. Surfman was an enlisted position, part of the lifesaving stations found along both coasts and the Great Lakes. The stations were small and usually consisted of a building with a boat launch. The surf-men were excellent at maneuvering the lifesaving rowboats in all types of rugged weather. The pay was sixty dollars a month. During the war, many surfmen saw action in the early landings in the Pacific because of their skills at handling small beach craft. I never mentioned the Coast Guard inter-view to my mother. A few weeks later she told me she received a phone call from the Coast Guard, looking for a John Merrill, and told them they had the wrong number. I guess she was a little surprised.

The day I enlisted in July 1938, I drove my 1937 Ford coupe to the Buffalo surf station. Once again, swimming helped me out in a new and unfamiliar situation. When queried about my swimming abilities, I displayed my skills and received immediate acceptance and identity with the crew.

Wherever I was stationed, I looked for the local YMCA and continued my swims. It was only in 1939, when I was transferred to Radio Operators' School at Fort Trumbull in

Connecticut, that swimming was a rare occurrence. Six months later I was sent to Boston, a transfer that implied sea duty in the North Atlantic. While there, I joined the Lynn YMCA swim team. One of the team members was a fellow by the name of Riley. Fifty years later we renewed our friendship and swam at a masters swim meet in California. In February 1940 I suffered an emergency appendectomy and was in the hospital for several weeks. I was not looking forward to spending my twenty-third birthday in a hospital ward, but things picked up when my Lynn swim coach appeared at the door with a birthday cake. In a place far from home, to be remembered was significant. And to be remembered by my swim coach just proves the point that swimming makes for good friends.

A three-year dry spell from swimming took place between 1941 to 1944. Those years and earlier during iceberg patrol in the North Atlantic, left me like a fish out of water. I was transferred down to Washington, D.C., for a twelve-month course at a civilian radio engineering school. Swimming was not included in this assignment. Upon graduation, I received orders for a secret assignment on Long Island while my newly married roommate received orders to Alaska. He was not happy. I intervened on his behalf and asked the officer in charge to switch our assignments so he could be with his wife. They agreed and I found myself in Alaska. By the way, that secret assignment on Long Island, turned out to be involved with making pre-invasion installations on Japanese-held islands in the Pacific. In contrast, Alaska—with no swimming and thirteen feet of rainfall each year—was no great switch for me. To adapt, I wrote a military update for the *Ketchikan Chronicle* and also wrote for another weekly, the *Alaska Fishing*

News. In the spring of 1944, I was transferred to the U.S. Coast Guard Radio Engineering and Maintenance School in Groton, Connecticut, to teach for the following seven years.

An opportunity to work at the U.S. Navy Underwater Sound Laboratory at Fort Trumbull in New London was brought to my attention, and after leaving the Coast Guard in 1951 I accepted a position at the laboratory as an electronic scientist. My main career until retiring in 1979 was at the laboratory primarily involved in electromagnetics, specifically as they relate to submarine radio communications.

I really shouldn't use the word *retired.* My interests in engineering, swimming, or writing did not falter with retirement. I've always held the belief that with reasonable health and modest fiscal independence, retirement gives us an opportunity to become what we really are. This postcareer period of my life provides me with the freedom and more time to do what I always enjoy, especially swimming. It removes me from the rigors of the day. In the pool I can concentrate on the stroke, the kick, and pacing, not on work and the realities outside the pool. You can't possibly be thinking about anything else if you want to be good at it. Especially with my specialty, the backstroke; if I'm not careful, I'll bump my head on the wall.

When I received my first invitation to swim in a USMS-sponsored meet in 1973, I was pleased. That same year I won my first USMS trophy for accumulating the most points at a New England regional meet and have competed every year in their events. After years of missing the competitive spirit of the sport, I found it again with renewed spirit.

Before joining the USMS I attended swim meets primarily as a spectator for my children, sometimes a meet official, and sometimes a coach. Watching them, I frequently thought how wonderful it would be for me to have the opportunity to compete again. With the USMS it has happened and now my days start out with a set of predawn calisthenics, followed by a short drive to Waterford High School for my daily workout, usually adding up to 1,500 meters, just shy of a mile. When I am training for a meet, I'll return later in the day for a second workout. My style in the pool is slow and steady. Some say it looks effortless, but believe me, it's not. A part of my workout is just kicking on my back. I do three hundred yards of kicking, five- to six-hundred yards freestyle, then a five-hundred-yard backstroke, and finally fifty yards of freestyle. A few weeks prior to competition, I'll increase my effort and routine. It's like a formula and it works for me. Each workout is recorded in my journal, which I have been keeping forever. It's more than just a journal of the workouts; it's an assessment of my efforts. If I am swimming outdoors, I'll make a special note of the weather (a happy face, or a frown). As I mentioned, my specialty is the backstroke, but I keep plugging away at the freestyle, always believing I've got plenty of time to improve.

Over the years, I realize I am slowing down at a pace of about one percent a year. It's ephemeral, the way it slips away. A half second here, a half second there, and it's gone. I realize I am not capable of cranking out the speedy times I recorded in past decades, but I have no remorse. With my background in technology, physics, and calculus, combined with my drive to always find a better way, I've made a kind of science out of my swimming. I guess you could say I swim smarter, not faster. I concentrate more on efficiency than power, and the clock I am beating is against myself, not a competitor. I've reached an age when I have to understand and face my limitations. I've tried other sports, but never took to them like my desire to swim. I used to ride my bike quite a bit and one time rode with my son back from Skidmore College, about two hundred miles. I also rode my bike to work here in New London. But swimming has always been my first love. It's all I've known. I love the meets, I love the people. Everyone cheers for everyone else, and afterward there is a picnic lunch we all partake in and recount the meet's events.

I swim every day and race several times a year in local, regional, and national meets sanctioned by U.S. Masters Swimming. My current age group is eighty to eighty-four, and sometimes I don't have any competition. Of course, that means I come in first, but I like to have some competition! Four times I've earned All-American status for recording the fastest time of the year in races for my age group. I am very proud of that, but what it all boils down to is luck. Life is a lot of luck. There are minefields out there, and if you're lucky you avoid stepping on them. I'm surrounded by my family, have a full schedule of research projects, and just recently we returned from a brief summer vacation with all the children at Squam Lake in New Hampshire. Every morning I'd get in a canoe and paddle out toward the middle of the lake and read the *New York Times*. I befriended a fellow who was ninety-two years old and was somewhat upset because he had just retired his car keys. He was still sharp as a tack and dressed very dapper. At a glance, you could tell he took care of himself and cared about his appearance. I want to be like him when I get old. I don't ever want to lose my desire to learn and know.

It's important to have an allegiance to places and things. That's what gives us our strong roots. I've always viewed my life as one big adventure that I hope never ends. Who knows? Maybe I'll go back to Buffalo for the next high school reunion.

ADVANTAGE: LIFE

VAL OROSZ

Born: 2-1-21

Residence: Saddle Brook,
New Jersey

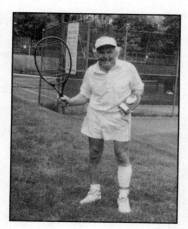

> **"I shall grow old, but never lose life's zest, because
> the road's last turn will be the best." —Henry Van Dyke**

*From the time he was a child, Val's life was dedicated to hard work
and family. The kids in his melting-pot neighborhood were judged
not by their accents or cultural ways but whether they could throw a
football. Tennis was considered a game for sissies. Years later, Val
watched a tennis match and told his wife it looked easy. She challenged his braggadocio, so he bought a cheap racquet, entered a tournament, and won. Tennis became his passion, his mental and
physical lifesaver. At seventy-eight, Val is still going strong on the tennis circuit. When asked the secret to his youthful aging and incredible
stamina on the court, he looks perplexed. He doesn't see himself as
different. However, the aging experts would most likely point to his
strong family roots, an active exercise program, and basically being
too busy to think about growing old as the keys to Val's contented life.*

I can't believe anyone would be interested in reading about
my life. I haven't done anything out of the ordinary. I didn't
even go to college, or graduate from high school for that

matter. Over the years I've gotten used to my lack of schooling, but I've never been ashamed of it. I have worked hard all my life, harder than most people I've ever met. But I will tell you one thing. When I step on the tennis court it doesn't matter what degree my opponent has or what ivy-covered institute he went to, I usually beat the pants off him.

I grew up in Garfield, the youngest of six kids, with my parents who immigrated from Hungary. We lived on a dead-end street where everyone was from another country, fresh off the boat at Ellis Island. It never mattered to any of us where we were from. The only thing that mattered is that we got along. There was always a pickup game of football, baseball, any sport. We took our sports very seriously and were always active. When I was fourteen I won first prize in a scooter contest and won a tennis racquet. Never did use that racquet; I think it just rotted away in my closet. My friends and I viewed tennis a sissy sport. However, I did love ping-pong and was very good at it. Maybe that's where I developed such strong hand-eye coordination.

I quit high school to go to work. We were very poor and felt at the time that making money was more important than an education. When I was eighteen, my father died of a heart attack. He was only fifty-six at the time. By then all six of us were out working to help support my mother.

My first job was at the local farms, picking crops or doing whatever was needed. A lot of boys in my area were just as poor, so there was stiff competition to get to the jobs early. Up at 5 A.M., I'd hop on my bike and make the rounds of farms in Clifton, Elmwood Park, Passaic, wherever I had to go. Sometimes I'd have to travel ten to twelve miles to get a job. We were paid ten to twenty cents an hour and put in ten-hour days. At the end of the day, I'd ride home and was so happy to be able to give my wages to my mom. After dinner she would hand me back four cents, and I'd run down to the corner store where we hung out and splurge on two ice pops. That was the best part of the day. Then I'd go to bed and start all over again the next morning. I didn't think of it as hard times; didn't really know I was poor. I had a very happy childhood. In the winter, when the farms closed up, I'd walk from saloon to saloon shining shoes. Most of the boys charged five cents a shine, but I'd say, "Pay me whatever you think it's worth." Sometimes that worked and I'd get ten to fifteen cents, and sometimes I'd get stiffed.

My favorite job was hanging around the corner gas station trying to learn how to repair cars. The owner, an old Italian guy who took a liking to me, occasionally let me do some menial work but he couldn't afford to pay me. He said he'd pay me in coffee and doughnuts. He'd tell me, "This is hard, dirty work, but if you learn to fix cars you'll always have a job." Over time I proved myself by doing anything that was asked of me, and eventually he hired me at $1.50 a day. I worked on Model A Fords, DeSotos, and other models from the 1930s and 40s. This was during the depression so even with this pay it was tough to make ends meet. At night, I'd unwind by playing pickup football games, which was pretty rough but all the kids got along. It's not like it is today where people are made to feel different. We all mixed. It didn't matter where someone came from. Everyone shared and contributed to the neighborhood in whatever way they could. A professional fighter, Tippy Larkin, lived near me and trained in his manager's garage. All the kids loved to watch him, and he was very good to us. He taught us the basics of boxing and conditioning, which I still use today.

When World War II broke out, I had to report to the draft board. I remember so vividly walking out of the house that day and down the street while my mother watched from our doorway. She never took her eyes off me until I was out of her sight. I could feel her eyes penetrating right through me. It must have been so hard on her. However, I was soon back after being deferred for curvature of the spine. I was always very short, about five foot five, due to a curve in my spine that got worse during a particularly rough football game. When I was fifteen a young doctor by the name of Henry Kessler performed experimental surgery on my back, taking a nine-inch bone from my left shin and fusing it to my spine. That young doctor went on to found the famous Kessler Institute for Rehabilitation. You'd think I'd have a tough time walking, not to mention playing pickup games, but it never stopped me.

In 1946 I married my Edna, the love of my life, and we moved in with her parents in a small apartment downstairs from them. They didn't want to charge us rent, but Edna insisted and sometimes she would raise the rent herself and give them more. My wife was a beautiful person and made me feel ten feet tall. She was my backbone. Edna and I had two sons, Gary and Tom, and I worked day and night to make ends meet. I eventually opened up my own garage in 1942 with my oldest brother. That partnership lasted three years until we had a falling-out. In 1945 I bought a dump truck and hired myself out, hauling anything from bricks to manure to produce. It was hard times but I wouldn't quit the day until I made some money. Two years later I bought another gas station, more a shack than anything else, right on Route 17 in Paramus with another partner. Route 17 was still mostly farmland at the time. We did everything in that garage; repaired cars and lawn mowers, sharpened tools, sold candy and cigarettes. Eventually Edna and I had the funds to move to our own house in Saddle Brook. The municipal tennis courts were across the street from our house and I'd watch those crazy fools in white shorts chasing tennis balls. I'd say to Edna, "Anyone can do that." She challenged me to enter a tournament so I bought three cheap racquets for the kids and me and signed us up. In my first tennis tournament ever, I won the men's open division and was instantly hooked. At forty years of age I found a new passion. I'll tell you, I think all those years of playing ping-pong helped my game. I never took a lesson, never had any real strokes, I just got to every ball and hit it back. If you want to know the real truth as to why I possibly could have won, I didn't want to have to tell Edna I'd lost.

By day I'd run the auto shop and at night play tennis. I'd be in my overalls at the garage, full of grease, and then quickly wash up and change in the bathroom and emerge in my tennis whites. I joined a club in Nutley and played all the time. After I was a member for over twenty-five years, they gave me a lifetime membership. But a few years later they wanted to cancel that and charge me again. I don't know why, maybe they thought it was a losing proposition and I would outlive them. Anyway, I didn't renew because by then I was playing at the Upper Ridgewood Tennis Club most of the time. I was so hooked on the game, I joined the tournament trail and played everywhere, mostly singles and on all types of surfaces. By the time I was fifty-five, I was ranked number three in the East for the men's fifty-five category. I was always the shortest player out there but usually ended up on the long end of the score.

I finally retired from the garage in 1984 when I was sixty-one. By that time my younger son Tom and my partner's son had been working with us and it was time to let go. I really didn't want to, but it was right to let the kids take over. I was becoming the old man hanging around thinking they were doing everything wrong, just because it wasn't the way I did it. God bless them, they are now doing better than I ever did. One day they were cleaning up the place and found an old box full of receipts from when we first opened in 1947. They couldn't believe what we charged people. Two dollars for this, three dollars for that. I tried to explain that we were hungry, that we had to undercut the competition, but they just laughed.

Anyway, one day Edna said to me, "Now that you are retired don't think you're going to sit around the house all day and rot. Let's buy an RV and travel." We bought our first van in 1985 and put on 74,000 miles. We had so much fun. We bought a second one in 1989 and that one had 94,000 miles before I sold it. I just bought my third van in August and I'm up to 17,000 already. We drove everywhere. I have friends in just about every state. Our son Gary is in Oregon and we drove there quite a bit. Some of these friends I only see once a year but we never miss a beat.

Edna loved the game and was very supportive. She would accompany me and sit on the sidelines, usually knitting, quietly listening to all the comments that were being made about my playing. One day a woman was commenting on my speed and agility and said, "Wow, look at that guy. I wonder what he eats. He must have a great diet to be in that kind of shape." Edna just looked up at her and said, "Junk food."

She died in 1990 of cancer and there isn't a day that goes by that I don't miss her. I wish I had spent more time with her than on the tennis court, but she loved to watch me play. Her passing put me in a tailspin and I couldn't get motivated, didn't even want to play tennis. I became despondent. My long-time doubles partner, Hank Conway, finally pulled me out of it by signing me up for some tournaments. I swear to God, tennis brought me back to life. I don't know what I would have done if I didn't have that stupid game to look forward to.

Hank and I make quite a pair. We teamed up twenty years ago after Hank watched me destroy a singles opponent during a league tournament. I was fifty-five at the time and my opponent was a college student. As Hank recalls, I left the kid hanging on the net. Hank and I play so well together. He has the best backhand-driving volley on the circuit. We move like one. In 1996 and 1997 we won the U.S. Tennis Association's (USTA) Men's 75s National Grass Court Championships at the Tennis Hall of Fame in Newport. It was a great moment. We won the title in straight sets, 6–4, 6–3. The next week we went on to win the National 75s Doubles Clay Court Championship in Arlington Virginia. President Clinton awarded us the USTA award, which is a gold tennis ball. By the end of 1996, Hank and I had been ranked number one in the country for seventy-five-and-over two years in a row. As much as I like to win, Hank's friendship means more to me than anything. We play hard and then enjoy needling each other in the locker room afterward. We can also battle each other across the net in singles and argue relentlessly over line calls.

As I look back on my life, I can't believe how lucky I've been. At an age when most of my peers are hobbling around with braces after hip and knee replacement surgery, I have never had a serious injury. Of course I ache afterward but nothing that will keep me off the courts. I attribute that to starting the game at forty instead of fourteen. I think that saved me. Some tennis players are not good athletes and it shows. They don't have the moves, the natural feel for it. Anyone who is a good athlete and takes a few lessons and gets plenty of playing time can get pretty good if they work at it. You also have to know when to change your strategy. The reason I can still beat some of those college guys who hit rockets at me from the baseline is my drop-dead drop shot. They hate it; it frustrates them. They feel they should have won, that they were the better player, but in the end I'm the one who wins. Hank and I won our club's men's 45s doubles tournament when we were seventy-five. That was a fun day. Everyone was cheering for the old guys. Strategy and patience will beat brute and brawn most times. The other key is wanting to win more than your opponent. That emotional edge is a killer. Some of my toughest competitors are seventy-five and eighty. They are so damn smart, even though a bit daft in the head. Sometimes their wives have to direct them onto the court, but once they know where they are, they kick in.

My seventy-nine-year-old sister lives with me now and although at first I wasn't sure of this arrangement, it seems to be working. She likes taking care of people and still drives her lady friends around wherever they need to go. She cooks and cleans, which I am not very good at. I don't see dust. Three months each winter I live in Florida and play the circuit down there. I drive down in my van, which makes the trip convenient and cost effective. Leaving Saddle Brook at 8 A.M., I drive till it gets dark and stop for a meal. Then I drive to midnight, when I'll pull over at a rest stop and sleep till the morning and continue the drive, arriving in Florida by noon the next day. I live in my van and use my bike to get where I need to go.

I don't know why I am able to do the things I do at seventy-eight, an age when most of my peers are either in nursing homes or have passed away. I worked hard all my life, raised two great sons and loved my wife. My family is still very important to me. A few times a year I drive out to Oregon to visit my son, who has built a beautiful home there. He even built a trophy room for me, where he keeps my awards and newspaper clippings. My other son lives nearby so I get to see him and spend time with my grandsons, teaching them tennis. My life is full. I'm not a rich man, far from it. But if I only had two nickels to rub together and my kids needed something, I'd give them both nickels. On the other side of the spectrum is a friend of mine who spends his days watching TV and drinking beer. He can't even see his feet through his big, fat stomach. I feel sorry for him. He gave up. You need something to love in life, whether it's a person, a sport, a hobby, whatever it is that gets you out of bed in the morning. I love the game of tennis. It makes me smile, and when I stop smiling I'll know it's over. Most of the tennis players I've had the pleasure to meet are terrific people. Of course there are a few jerks out there, but I stay away from them. I have found in my forty years of playing that the personality you see on the court is the real personality of the person. If they are nasty on the court, they are nasty in life and vice versa. I am never disrespectful on the court. I'm just happy to be there. I have so many lifelong friends from this game, I don't even bother with shaking hands anymore; I go directly for the hug.

Most anyone can have what I have if they work at it. And

having a positive attitude definitely makes everything in life easier. When I am in Florida, I stay with a friend whose wife had a very bad stroke, which left her paralyzed and unable to speak or walk. Lee spends her days in a wheelchair but despite her disabilities, this beautiful lady is always cheerful and fun to be with. We spend our evenings doing hundred-piece puzzles together. She struggles with each piece, painstakingly trying to fit them. You should see the smile on her face when she gets a piece in. It brightens up the room.

Every night before bed I say my prayers, talk with Edna, and look forward to the next day when I wake up and thank God for making it through the night. I still feel needed. I have a reason to go on.

SOUTHERN CHARM

LUCILLE SINGLETON

Date of birth: 9-18-23

Residence: New York City

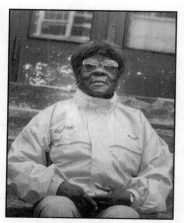

"The heads of strong old age are beautiful beyond all grace of youth." —Robinson Jeffers

People like Lucille don't come by often and when they do, you want to embrace them, stay close to them, be their friend and learn from them. Lucille has led a hard life, more different and difficult than most. But she has a way of looking only at the goodness life has brought, and feeling blessed and fortunate. As a child she worked on a plantation in the South, eventually working her way north, leaving family and friends behind. Thinking that running would be good exercise she joined the New York Road Runners Club and volunteered for years before entering her first road race at sixty-seven and her first marathon at seventy-five. When she retired from housekeeping, she got bored and became a construction worker, winning praise for her strong work ethic, and the affectionate on-site nickname, Grandma. Lucille is a no-nonsense woman who plans to run maybe just one more marathon and build maybe just a few more buildings before retiring, yet again.

I'm from a little place called Philips, South Carolina, but I never did like it much so I tell people I'm from Charleston.

Philips had these creepy little caterpillars all over the ground and I just didn't take a liking to those bugs, couldn't wait to leave. My family worked on the Huntington Hartford Plantation down there. Mother was the cook, I washed the dishes and did general cleanup, and my father was the manager of the plantation. We had a strong work ethic from the start. I did my job after school, which was right across the street. My mom was a great cook. Her fried chicken was famous and we made dressing—not stuffing—from scratch. I still use her corn dressing recipe and my grandkids love it. My two older sisters also worked at the plantation and then had to take care of our house. Since I was the baby, I got away with not doing a lot of chores.

I never did travel much although I wanted to leave Philips all my life, couldn't wait for the day when I would just pack up and go. Made it to Florida once, on a plane but that was so scary for me I never did get on one again. I was all right until they said to buckle the seat belt. I kept wondering, If we are gonna be safe, why do I need this seat belt? And then when they started talking about a life jacket, that did it. Heck, there won't be enough time to even put it on if the plane is going down. It didn't seem natural so I never did fly again.

I married at twenty-seven; it was good at the start but soon unraveled. I will say he was a good father to our three children, but our relationship wasn't and we separated. Money was an issue, as there wasn't much coming in. Even with work, he was only making two dollars a week, and then he got sick with high blood pressure and couldn't work at all. I knew I had to get a decent job to support the family but there were no good-paying jobs down there. Desperate and with no alternative, I made the decision to come north for work, which meant leaving my children behind with their father. Our local newspapers carried ads from employment agencies up north looking for child-care domestics. I responded to one and traveled by bus to New York. I went straight to the agency and sat in the reception area waiting to be claimed by a family. It was so nerve-racking just sitting there wondering who would come through the door and take me home with them. All these girls just like me sitting there. We had no idea what destiny had in store. When they called my name, I went to another room where a family with two small children was waiting to evaluate me. As I entered, it seemed as if heaven lit up. The little boy took one look at me and said, "Oh Mommy, I want this one!" I lived with them for four years. In fact, we still keep in touch. It was a wonderful job with a wonderful family. God sure did look down on me that day.

Although the job was a blessing, my life was so hard without my children. It was just something I had to do and they were the sacrifice. I sent all my money back home to the children. For four years I never had one dime to call my own. Even on my days off, I cleaned houses for other people. But I was lucky because the family I worked for invited my kids to stay with them during the summers. They were so generous to me and the kids. We had great family reunions during the summers but I missed them all the more come August. It's a terrible thing for a mother to be pulled apart from her children but for me it was the only way to ensure that they survived.

After four years of being a live-in, I decided it was time for a change so I moved in with my aunt and took all sorts of jobs to continue making as much money as I could. I did everything and anything, from factory jobs to housecleaning to caretaking and cooking for the elderly. I finally made enough money to get a place of my own and bring my children up to live with me. By now my daughters were in high school and the change was easy for them. But my son didn't come at first. I love my son dearly and missed him so much, but he said to me, "No, Mom, you were up north for so long while Dad took care of us. He is very sick and I won't leave him now that he needs me." I understood. That's his nature. He is a very good boy. Things were much easier having my daughters. They got jobs baby-sitting and things finally seemed to be just fine. But I guess my life was just meant to be hard. My younger daughter died when she was just nineteen. We had only been reunited a short few years when blood pressure complications took her from me. I tried everything to get her to change her diet and try to be healthy but she was stubborn and in the end I lost her. My mother died of high blood pressure so it does run in my family. It was terrible times, but you just have to pick yourself up and go on.

By now my husband had died and my son joined us in New York. We all moved into an apartment on 112th Street, right next door to where I live now. And my son now owns the building. But to continue my story, it's now the 1970s and I was taking care of an old woman whose granddaughter would come visit. The granddaughter was a runner, and it made me remember how much I loved to run back home. Of course I don't mean on a team or anything, there was nothing like that. But me and my girlfriends just loved to run down those long roads feeling the wind in our hair and seeing who could go the fastest. And that was always me. I was the leader; I won all the races. Looking back on those days I can see that even then I was always determined, usually got what I wanted if I tried hard enough. Wasn't ever a quitter. Anyway, I got the desire to run again after seeing the granddaughter so I asked her what should I do to start running. She suggested I join the New York Road Runners Club so in 1979, at the age of fifty-six, I became a member. But I never did run the races. I became a volunteer and worked the races instead of running. I'd be at the races at 5:30 setting up and stay till it was over and tear it down. I'd do any job, but I didn't like the water stations in the winter. Too cold and messy. I did run on my own but was too intimidated to run a race, thought I'd be last and I didn't want to be last. You couldn't get me to run a four-mile, five- or six-mile race. Not me. I was afraid. But yet I got up every morning at 3:30 and ran four miles up Eighth Avenue. That may sound crazy, but it fits my schedule. The alarm goes off at 3:30, I have myself a cup of coffee and juice, dress in light colored clothing, and head up Eighth Avenue. I used to run down Eighth instead but it works better for me to run up so I can see any traffic heading my way. I run in the middle of the street so it is important for me to be able to see oncoming traffic, although at that hour I have the road to myself. And it's not that dark, as the streetlights shine pretty bright. That's why I like running in the middle of the street. After a few weeks everybody got to know me and we would wave at each other. The bus drivers and policemen look out for me. If I take a few days off, they get worried and ask around to make sure I'm all right.

For eleven years I plodded on with my own running schedule and worked the races. When I started working the New York City Marathon, I was amazed at all these people running such a long time. I love working that race. Usually I am the first person at setup and the last person at takedown. And in between I work the Expo Center, handing out the race numbers and T-shirts to the runners. They are always so excited. I got to wondering what it would be like to actually run the marathon. Then I started to say, "Someday I am going to do that." You can't help but want to run when you see the excitement. Finally I took the plunge and entered my first road race, a three-mile run, in 1990 when I was sixty-seven. I was scared but I finished, and not in last place! It made me realize I could do it. That was a big breakthrough for me and I continued running short-distance races. To this day I still look over my shoulder to see if I am in last place and need to run faster. I don't ever want to be last. Taking up running was the first time in my life I did something just for myself. And you know what? It felt good. I had been neglecting myself and my health for so long I couldn't believe how simple it really was to just get up one day and do it. I bought a pair of running shoes, read a book on how to stretch and run correctly, and that was it. Truly, it's the best part of my day.

In 1992 the lady I was taking care of for the past several years moved to Florida, and instead of looking for another job I decided to quit. For two years I didn't do anything. I became a couch potato. Still did my morning run, but then came home and sat. Finally I decided to move myself off the couch and get a job. Heck, I was seventy years old and not ready to give up living. Not wanting to go back to domestic housework, I went to an employment agency to seek a job. When the lady saw how old I was, she said, "What you want a job for now? You're too old to work. Go home." But I said I wanted to work and she said she'd look but I never did get a call from her. So I figured it was up to me to get my own job. I knew I wanted something different, so I walked around the neighborhood looking for opportunities. I saw construction sites and thought, Why not? One day I got the nerve up to speak to a flag girl on a local construction site and she told me to call her uncle, who was the foreman on the site. So I called him and he gave me a very hard time but that didn't stop me. I was determined to get this job, and finally he agreed to see me. We met at the site and he said, "I have a job for you. Stay here and another guy named John will come by and give you the job." Well, when John came by he didn't talk to me, didn't even look at me. Finally I had to say I was waiting for him to give me a job and he said, "I don't have anything for you. Go home." That night I called the foreman back and told him John wouldn't give me a job and he told me to come back the next day. When I got to the site, John was there looking angry at me and brought me to the basement of the site, where garbage and rubbish were piled high to the ceiling. John told me my job was to clean out the room. At first, I was going to refuse. I was sick of cleaning up other people's mess and didn't want to start my new career cleaning. But I bit my lip, took the garbage bags that John was holding out, and cleaned that room up so fast your head would spin.

That next week, when I reported for another job, John said he didn't need me. But the foreman knew how much I wanted to work so he introduced me to another contractor around the corner on a job that was just starting and he told me to come back in two weeks. But I didn't want to wait so I showed up the next day. I went every day and just stood around waiting. The last day of the first week, he let me work. They were doing demolition and they were somewhat worried it would be too dangerous but I hung in there, said I would do any job they asked of me. Well, I spoke too soon, but once again bit my lip. My first job was walking across those tiny little beams way up high bringing supplies to the guys. They taught me how to walk on beams so I wouldn't fall. As I took my first steps across I said, "Lord have mercy. How am I ever going to do this?" But I did and ended up working nineteen jobs with that contractor. After I proved myself, all the guys loved me. Call me Grandma. They're good to me because I do what I'm told and I do a good job. Sometimes when I'm walking down the street and a truck of workers go by that I've worked with, they jump out and give me a hug. Most people can't believe I started a new career at seventy—and then they really go nuts when they learn my new career is in construction.

I've been doing construction going on six years now and I love it. Mostly I do carpentry and plumbing. I know my limits and stick with what I know. Don't work with the heavy equipment or machinery. When I report to a new job, I don't wait for anyone to tell me what to do. I just start working. Meanwhile the other guys are standing around waiting for the foreman to give them assignments. When he gets on the job he says, "Why are you guys just standing around waiting? Look at Lucy over there. I never have to tell her what to do." Construction has been the best thing that ever happened to me. I still get up at 3:30, do my four-mile run, come home, shower, and get to work by 7 A.M. If I'm not working, I'll go back to bed after my run and sleep until noon and then clean my apartment or do errands, take my bike and go grocery shopping. Never did learn to drive. My favorite pastime is hanging out with the guys at the corner barbershop. We can talk about nothing all day. It's good times. We meet every day and if I don't show up, they come looking for me. They love to tease me about being old. But I tell them, "Don't go telling my bosses I'm old, 'cause I'm not."

I get a kick out of people's reactions to my career. When I go to cash my paycheck, the cashiers don't believe it's my check. The best fun is when I board a bus in my construction outfit—work boots, tool belt, hard hat—and then pay the senior citizen half fare. It really throws the bus drivers for a loop. They don't know what part of me to believe. I feel blessed to have this job. I earned it, I worked hard to get it, and stay fit to keep it. But I have to believe the mental and emotional strength to keeping this job comes from God.

My neighbors tell me I am an inspiration to Harlem. Everyone on the street greets me warmly. The only exception, which to this day makes me cry, is the one time in my life I was stopped by the police. I was reporting to a new job site and had to call my boss for the location. I dialed his beeper number and was waiting for him to call back when two policemen came up to me and asked what was I doing. I tried to explain but they started searching my bag and accusing me of dealing drugs. Of course they didn't find anything, but I was so humiliated and upset I just cried and cried. I'd never had a run in with the police, and here I was a seventy-one-year-old employed grandmother just trying to get to work. Later on when I told my friends about it, they said that particular corner where I was waiting was known as a drug dealer haven. I guess waiting for the phone was reason enough for the police to search me, but I will never forget that day.

After nineteen years of volunteering at the New York City Marathon, I decided to run it. So at seventy-five years old, I ran the marathon. Didn't train, don't like running distance, but I did it. It took me eight hours and two minutes. When I was at the start and saw that long expanse of the Verrazano

Bridge, the first two miles of the race, I started to look for a subway. I said to myself, "Lord have mercy, this is gonna be a long way home. I don't think I'll make it." I actually walked across the bridge. I truly would have taken a subway if I found one. Because of my years volunteering, everybody knew me and was very supportive. I ran with a friend from the runners club named Alison and everyone told her, "Don't cross the finish line without Lucille." She coached me the entire way. And everywhere I went I got hugs. Every water station, every aid station, even the runners on the course were coming over to give me hugs. For nineteen years I have seen the same faces, handed them T-shirts, put them on the bus to the start and many of them came back and remembered me. Now they saw me running and they wanted to help me. They gave me so many hugs. Crossing the finish line was the best moment in my entire life. I carried two red pom poms with me throughout the race so people could see me coming and when I got close to the finish line I raised those pom poms, shook them for all I was worth and let out a yell. About two hundred volunteers lined the finish line and greeted me. I cried like a baby.

And I wasn't last. In fact, as I was getting all this attention, I heard two women behind me saying, "Who does she think she is, getting all this attention?" The next day I went out and got my medal engraved. But the following day when I did the wash and put my NEW YORK CITY MARATHON FINISHER shirt in the dryer, someone stole it. I was so upset, but the club gave me another one.

I plan to run another marathon in 2000. But I'll train for that one. You know, it's sometimes discouraging when I'm out running and I'll see someone my age or close to it and they down me, discourage me. They say, "You're too old to run. Why don't you act your age?" Well you know what I say? If you want to be old, you make yourself old. Sometimes I'd come home crying because old people made me feel so badly. But I learned to get over that. And it's funny, but at my construction jobs no one makes fun of me. They respect me. And I do get a lot of requests from younger people to come and speak with their parents who don't do anything to stay healthy. They think I will be an inspiration. I'm honored they think so highly of me, but I am basically a shy person and don't like speaking in public. After I ran the marathon, I was asked to give a speech at the awards ceremony in front of thousands of people and all I could think of to say was, "I am Lucille Singleton, one of your grunts. I want to thank everyone who was worried about me running my first New York City Marathon." Not a bad speech.

I've always gone after what I want in life. Nobody I know is handing out things on a silver platter. There is no easy way out. I find that a lot of people are just lazy. They don't want to work hard for things; they prefer to sit around and complain when things don't go their way. I know there are people my age, and younger, who resent me for being so active and enjoying life. Maybe they're jealous but they only have themselves to blame. I wouldn't be jealous of them; I'd be supportive and proud of anyone who had the courage and determination to go after their dreams. When I went for that first construction job, I covered up this old gray head with a kerchief, trying to disguise my age. I found out most of the men had gray hair, too. We all get old. I just don't act it.

I run about two races a month, three-milers, and always win my age group. But that's not why I run; in fact most of the time I don't even stick around for the results. When I get back home there's usually a message saying, "Lucy, you won again. Come back and pick up your medal." When I go back down south for family reunions I bring my medals and they are so proud of me. This year I'll have five medals to show them. I'm very happy enjoying my life as it comes. I see a long life ahead of me.

A 79-YEAR-OLD CLASSIC

NONA TODD

Date of birth: 11-10-20

Residence: Bismarck,
North Dakota

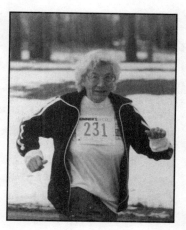

"As a white candle in a holy place, so is the beauty of an aged face." —Joseph Campbell

Nona is a class act. Has been her entire life. A legend among those who attend the Senior Olympics, Nona was not always an outstanding athlete. An automobile accident in 1982 left her in debilitating pain from severe, near-crippling arthritis. The doctors advised her not to walk and prescribed painkillers. But gutsy Todd said the heck with that and found walking to be her salvation. At sixty-eight, she entered the world of long-distance walking and became a race walker. Exercise is part of her everyday routine and she encourages her children, sixteen grandchildren and seven great-children to join her. When Nona is not race walking or attending the Senior Olympics, she can be found working on her farm. There are just not enough hours in the day for this lady.

There must be a connection between the way I entered this world and my feisty personality. I wasn't just delivered; I stormed into this world on the tails of one of the worst blizzards of the season with only my father and seven-year-old sister, Ruth, attending. Living on a ranch, my cowboy father had delivered calves and other animals but never his own child. He instructed my sister to boil water and sterilize utensils and the two of them brought me into this world. Afterward, he left Ruth to supervise our care while he hitched the horse and buggy to drive two and a half miles to fetch the local nurse. Fighting through drifts of snow that in some places towered over him, he returned four hours later with the nurse, who complimented him on a job well done. My birth certificate lists my dad as the attending physician and Pleasant View Ranch as my place of birth. That is my humble beginning to an incredible life.

Growing up on the ranch with eight siblings was hectic, with all of us assigned chores at tender ages. By the time I was four years old I was milking the cows, feeding the hogs, geese, ducks, and turkeys, carrying buckets of coal and water to the house, and helping with the canning and drying of the fruits and vegetables which had to last through the winter months. We made the thirty-mile trip to town by horse and buggy three times a year for supplies. We didn't own a car or have electricity or indoor bathrooms till much later in my life. With a hundred horses to tend, along with the cattle and gardens, there was plenty of work for everyone. It sounds hard, and it was, but I loved it. I learned to ride a horse before I could walk. My dad, Dick Dickenson (known to all as Rattlesnake Pete), was well known throughout the area, and along with taking care of our ranch he was called upon to train other horses and ride broncos on the rodeo circuit.

We were educated in a one-room schoolhouse that we attended for eight years with the same teacher, Mr. John Kinney. During the harsh winter months when the temperatures plummeted to fifty below, Dad improvised a taxicab on sleds. We'd heat rocks and flatirons and wrap them in blankets to keep us warm during the four-mile trip. Most of the time, though, we walked the distance—a total of eight miles in a day. Afterward, there was no time for rest or play, as the chores were waiting. Once in a while we'd get to ride the horses to school, three or four of us bouncing along on one horse, but Dad was stingy with his horses so he encouraged our walking.

After eighth grade my sister and I wanted to go to high school but that was in Carson, thirty miles from the ranch. We had to board, which my parents couldn't afford. Being resourceful folk they called upon their longtime friend, the governor of North Dakota. He was able to find housing and financing for my sister, but I was on my own. I managed to find a place to stay in exchange for caring for the landlady's seven children before and after school.

This was in the 1930s and everyone was feeling the effects of the depression. My sister and I went back home to help out, but the ranch suffered. There were no crops and the livestock, which we couldn't afford to feed anymore, had to be sold. Dad joined the Workman's Public Administration, which provided a bare existence, but time was our enemy and the ranch went bankrupt. The day we left, Dad packed all our belongings, took whatever horses were left, and as we silently and painfully drove away in the Model T Ford, he never once looked back.

Three days and 135 miles later, we reached our new life in Sterling, North Dakota. The two-room home stretched its seams to hold the ten of us. All of us had to earn our keep. I hired out at a neighboring farm milking twelve cows by hand, doing all the outside yardwork and some housework, all for $2.25 a week. I managed to do all of this at the same time as attending high school all day and working on my own farm, canning five hundred quarts of fruits, vegetables, and meat products for the winter. All three of my brothers were off fighting in the war, which made it difficult for my parents to keep up with the work, plus their health was failing. It was a very bleak time for us. The U.S. Government finally released one of my brothers from war duty to come home and help out. This was the only life I knew. There was no extra time or money for small pleasures but I had my family, I had responsibilities, and I knew from firsthand experience what it took to survive in this world.

In 1942 I graduated from high school and continued doing my chores back at the farm. My brothers had returned from the war, all intact except for one who lost an arm. My brother Bob introduced me to a war buddy, Roy Erickson, and a few months later we were married. I was nineteen years old. We bought our own farm, 320 acres, and worked side by side in the fields. We couldn't afford any help, so when I got pregnant I continued to work up to the delivery, and soon after I returned from the hospital I was back on the tractor. Seven kids later, and having to take in my parents, we had four generations of family living in our house. As if things weren't difficult enough, my dad died of a heart attack the day after he rounded up five hundred head of cattle as a favor to a neighbor. His loss was hard on me; he was the one who always held things together. A year later my husband died of a severe brain tumor, leaving me with seven children, aged seven months to seventeen years. I hardly knew night from day, as there was work for every minute. The care of the farm and the medical bills finally took their toll. I was so far in debt, the only thing to do was get deeper into debt. As my dad always said, you don't get nothing from nothing, so I bought a tavern twenty-three miles away. The younger children stayed home and worked the farm while the older ones helped me at the tavern. On a good night, I managed four hours' sleep.

My gambling paid off in the long run. And a small miracle helped. Interstate 94 was being built and as it came across North Dakota, the route was situated close to my café and bar. For four years I fed the construction crew and was able to pay off all my loans. I ran the tavern until 1976 when I decided to retire, but not before the state of North Dakota named me Bartender of the Year. By the time I retired, I had put in enough running, walking, and weight training between the ranch work and tavern to outdo a lifetime of sports events. It took its toll on my legs, as I needed three varicose vein operations and was told to stay off my feet. No chance of that happening in my lifetime.

As part of my retirement, I went on a long-awaited vacation to Hawaii. On the trip I met a man who a year later became my second husband. I was fifty-nine years old and starting another life. Ellis loved to travel and I visited places I never dreamed of seeing. We also got into hiking and he taught me to swim. But then another disaster struck my life. I had an automobile accident, leaving me crippled with severe pain in my legs, hips, and back. The doctors advised me not to walk. I spent most of my time in pain centers, hospitals and therapy. I had trouble going two or three steps. After years of no progress, I was so sick and tired of being on pain medication that I just got fed up and one day flushed all my medication down the toilet. I found a new doctor at the Mayo Clinic in

Arizona who told me to start swimming and walking as soon as possible. This was my second miracle.

My niece, who is only seven years younger than me, encouraged me to walk every day. Short walks became longer walks. We spent a lot of time in the pool and Jacuzzi. The doctor was very supportive of exercise therapy and encouraged it. Actually, he was instrumental in getting me to enter my first race, something I never thought possible. I completed my first race, a one-mile race walk, and he was there to cheer me on. I never thought I'd run or even walk any distance again, and here I was at sixty-two years old beginning to compete in a new sport. A horizon was open, but yet another tragedy was about to strike. My second husband died of multiple myeloma. He helped me all through my rehabilitation; he was so supportive and nurturing, and I missed him terribly. Thank God I had something new in life to help overcome my grief.

I became addicted to race walking. These old bones do hurt, but race walking is not as hard on the joints as running. The car accident caused severe arthritis in my joints, but I am sure that race walking is actually helping me deal with it. It keeps me agile and moving—good therapy for arthritic conditions. Sure, my ankles swell after a race but I work daily to ensure that I master my arthritic condition so it doesn't master me. The bottom line is that the benefits outweigh the negatives. It's far better than just sitting in a chair and hurting. I did too much of that while I was on the pain medication. I've been there and I'm not going back to that place. You tend to grow lazier by the day and think that things will never be as they were. But that's not true. I am proof that you can turn things around, and exercise is one of the ways. I have logged over 14,000 miles race walking and have over 786 awards and medals since 1988. Some of my most prized treasures are being named Athlete of the Year by the North Dakota Prairie Rose State Games in 1994 (a plaque with my picture and commentary hangs in the North Dakota State Hall of Fame), being named Athlete of the Year by the South Dakota State Games in 1995, and the Best Sport and Most Friendly Award from the Arizona State Games in 1996. In 1999 I received the Senior Award from the Arizona Governor's Council on Health, Physical Fitness and Sports. And I am proud to say I am a three-time winner of the Desert Shadows Trailer Park Shuffleboard Championship. Did I mention that I am also a billiard shark?

Somewhere along the line, older people begin to lose their confidence and become withdrawn. They turn to the radio or television, talk to telephone solicitors as a distraction, anything to keep them entertained. Even common household chores become drudgery. One phrase I commonly hear is, "Oh, I could never do that." People make up excuses not to exercise. I've heard them all. They make no attempt to participate in anything that will raise their heart rate. They become sedentary. If I didn't exercise, especially after the accident, I would have lost all my mobility and strength. In fact, I started simple exercises while just sitting in the chair.

The National Senior Olympic Games is one of the best organizations for seniors to get involved in sports. And don't let the title fool you. No one has to be of Olympic stature to participate. I have attended all the national games since 1989 and plan to keep attending until I can't walk anymore. At the state level I compete in race walking, javelin and discus throw, shot put, running long jump, 50-meter freestyle swim, horseshoes, eight-ball pool and many more events. This July I participated in a four-generation relay event at the North Dakota Prairie Rose State Games that included myself; my daughter Arlene, fifty-six; my granddaughter Lisa, thirty-two; and great-granddaughter Ashtyn, six years old. Family exercise and participation in events has been an ambition of mine. It is something we can all do together; something that binds families in a caring, fun partnership. I praise the Lord every day for such a great healthy relationship with my family. It's also other people I meet that make these events worthwhile. I have met wonderful gals and guys and have enjoyed their friendship throughout the years.

One of my favorite pastimes is speaking with children about exercise and aging. I sponsor Walk-Talk Days at the junior high school here in Bismarck. The students and I walk about three miles and I talk about my life and they get to ask me questions. It's a learning opportunity for all of us. I tell them, "It's not how old you grow, but how you grow old." More importantly, we bridge the gap between young and old and I become a positive role model for them. Their thank-you notes summarize what they learned from the experience. One student put it this way: "I want to be like you when I get old."

For me, there's just not enough time in the day to get everything accomplished. I like it that way.

JUST KEEP MOVING

EMMA "SIS" WARNKE

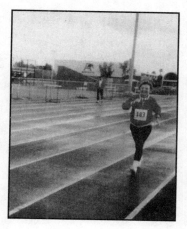

Date of birth: 4-22–18

Residence:
Las Cruces, New Mexico

"Wrinkles should merely indicate where the smiles have been." —Mark Twain

A self-described go-getter, Sis Warnke is living proof of the positive effects of exercise on the aging process. Sis never sits still. She took up running and biking at age sixty-two and has more medals, trophies, and awards than a gymful of people half her age. It is obvious that Sis derives enormous amounts of pleasure from being the grandma on the go. She had a knack for turning tasks into pleasant and rewarding experiences throughout her life—a positive outlook that goes hand in hand with her alertness and physical abilities. She is proud of the fact that she hasn't missed a Senior Olympic competition since the games were initiated in 1987. Sis sent me a package of her press clippings, and the first thing I noticed was her smile. In every snapshot, whether running a race or biking across the finish line, Sis is smiling. And it is a beautiful smile. It is obvious she loves her life.

Yesterday morning I ran in a track meet at the high school, participating in the 100-meter, 200-meter, 400-meter, 800- and 1,500-meter events. That afternoon I drove fifty miles into

Texas to another track meet, participating in the same events. Same races, same day, two different states. Not bad for an eighty-one-year-old lady.

I wasn't always so active and competitive. I grew up in Missouri (pronounced Miss-ara) with two older brothers. My parents never owned a car, preferring their horse and buggy. Eventually the twentieth century caught up with us and my older brothers pooled their money and bought a Model T Ford. In those days you didn't need a driver's license. If you could afford a car and could drive it, that was all the requirements needed. Females rarely drove. It was unheard of. I didn't drive till I got out of college.

We lived in Jefferson City, the capital. It was a beautiful place but had very cold winters and was hilly. As a kid, I walked to school—two miles, mostly uphill. Winters could be frigid and sometimes on my way to school I would have to thaw out at the post office.

After school there was no television, only chores like feeding the chickens. When the chores were done, I'd go inside and turn on the radio and listen to *The Adventures of Jack Armstrong, All American Boy*. It was a great show and I was hooked; tried not to miss a single adventure.

Graduating from high school, I wanted to attend college but it was the depression and my family had no money. I applied for a scholarship and received a grant for one year at Central Missouri State and loved it. I was determined to continue my college education and desperately sought other avenues of financing. The government sponsored a work program for twenty-five cents an hour and I signed up. For the next three years I worked and put all the money towards college, which left me nothing to live on. There were times I went hungry, but I had made up my mind to get a college degree and sacrificed everything for it. People everywhere were in the same boat. My neighbors ate nothing but beans and potatoes for dinner every night. When Dad lost his job my mother had to look for work. She had very nice handwriting and got a job at the State Board of Health writing birth certificates. While she was there she checked up on all of our birth certificates but mine wasn't listed. According to the state of Missouri, I wasn't born! Back then we were all birthed at home and the doctor was supposed to file a birth certificate. I guess the doctor failed to record it, so my mom wrote out my birth certificate. I still have it today. It's quite unusual to have a birth certificate written in your mother's handwriting.

At the advent of World War II my brothers were too old for the draft so we didn't have the heartache of sending sons overseas. However, I was dating a guy who did get drafted. Merlin was an only child from a small town in the Ozarks and we were in love. But he was soon shipped off to war with a promise to come home for me. He was stationed throughout Africa and Italy with the 34th Division and was one of the few survivors. I still have the letters he wrote to me. While he was off fighting, I graduated from college and acquired a job teaching physical education at a small Catholic high school in Illinois. It was a girl's boarding school and I lived in a one-room rental in a house near the school. I had a bike that I rode back and forth to school. Although we wrote faithfully to each other, communicating by letter was a slow process, so I never received word that he was coming home on a two-week furlough. One night I took my bike out to visit a friend at the same time Merlin had acquired his two-week pass and was on his way to see me. When he reached my house, he was told I was out for the evening. When he explained who he was, the owners of the house gave him an extra bike, and off he went in search of me. It was late as I was riding home and saw a man on a bike on the wrong side of the road and thought, What a crazy fool. Then that fool started to cross the street heading directly towards me and it wasn't till the last second that I realized it was Merlin! I hadn't seen him in four years but our love was still strong and two weeks later we were married. He moved into my little one-room rental and we had ourselves a two-week honeymoon. When he was scheduled to report back, we said a tearful good-bye and off he went but instead of being shipped back, he received news that the war was over. We lived in that one-room bedroom until my school contract was finished in June.

By 1959 we had four kids and started to move around a bit looking for the right place to settle. After fifteen years of teaching in Illinois and withstanding the cold, bitter winters we wanted a better and warmer place to live and found it in Las Cruces, New Mexico. After the ice and snowstorms of Illinois winters, the year-round warm weather was very inviting. We both ended up teaching in the same district, me at the middle school and Merlin at the high school. For the next twenty years, we lived a wonderful life. Merlin taught drivers' education and coached track and golf while I coached volleyball, basketball, softball and track. In thirteen of my nineteen years my seventh, eighth and ninth grade teams swept the annual city meet championships. None of my teams ever finished lower than third place.

Then life twisted. In 1976, three years short of Merlin's planned retirement, he died of liver cancer at fifty-seven.

Once he was diagnosed, he lived another six months. Now I was a widow with four children to put through college. You don't expect things like that in life. He was the only man I ever loved, and his death was devastating to the kids and me. But life goes on. I couldn't bury myself in grief, let it drag me down. My kids were great during this time; I don't think I could have managed without their support. For seventeen years my only focus was work, the kids, and making sure each one of them got through college. Merlin would have been so proud of them. They all became teachers. Finally, in 1979, I retired at age sixty-two.

Now that I had a life of my own, no kids at home, and plenty of time, I wanted to do something just for me. I didn't want to sit down in that rocking chair and never get up. I wanted to start living again. I knew it would be a sport of some kind that would keep me going, but didn't want to be tied down to something that was too complicated or where I needed a partner or lots of equipment like golf or tennis. That boiled down to running, so one day I just stepped out the door and went on my first run. Some people say they are too old to run, but I didn't feel that way. Never having run before, I didn't know if I could do it, so I started out slowly. I counted every step and each day increased my steps. By the end of the first month I was up to one mile. During this time I also opened up a dancewear shop in conjunction with my daughter Michelle's dance studio. She had been a physical education teacher and dance instructor at Mayfield High School and was making the transition to full-time dance instructor. A few days after I retired she came and asked me what my plans were. I told her my first priority was to finally clean out the garage. She said "Fine. When you finish that, how would you like to open a dancewear shop?"

My store flourished and also became the meeting place for members of the Bike and Chowder Club, which started up in 1983 as a way for anyone from eighteen to eighty to get together and enjoy a bike ride. We go out for an early-morning twenty-mile ride three times a week and then "chow down" to a big breakfast; thus the name Bike and Chowder Club. In 1980, a year after I retired, I started feeling my energetic oats and began entering races. No spring chicken, I was in the sixty-to-sixty-five age division and to my surprise there was some good competition. I loved competing, something I felt I never had the opportunity to do growing up. Even after all those years of coaching, I never got to do it for myself. So this was fun! Running and cycling became my passions.

Four years later, at age sixty-five, I was beating my competition. All it takes is a little bit of willpower. I realized I felt better closing in on seventy than I ever did at fifty-five. Once you pass fifty-five, you age pretty fast if you don't stay active. While scanning the newspaper one morning, I saw an announcement looking for senior citizens interested in running. This was the beginning of the local competition for the state Senior Olympics. I entered and qualified in the 50-yard dash, 100-yard dash, 440-yard run, and one-mile run. I tried to run in just about every race that came along. That year, 1984, I won twelve gold medals at the New Mexico Senior Olympics and my new career was launched.

By age seventy-five I was a regular on the race circuit and was referred to in the local papers as "Young at Heart, An Inspiration." When I attended events where people didn't know me, they would take one look at this old body and expect me to crawl across the finish line. But I never did. In fact, I was beating people in the forty- and fifty-year age groups. My kids gave me a huge seventy-fifth birthday surprise party that year, complete with a five-tier cake, and a swing band that played all the big band hits from my era. I think I danced every dance. It was a night I will never forget. My date was my biking buddy and boyfriend, Bob Seidel. We had been courting for some time and although I never thought I could fall in love again after being married to such a wonderful first husband, I found myself falling in love all over again. Seven days after my fabulous party, in April 1993, we got married. Bob and I do everything together. He attends the Senior Olympics with me, participating in cycling, bowling, and horseshoes. We are both very lucky to have found each other and are having a great life. We never seem to come down with illnesses or suffer any major injuries.

At age seventy-nine I competed in the 1,500-meter run and the 40K cycling race at the U.S. Senior Sports Classic in Tucson, Arizona. I did every event I could squeeze in. Now that I am in the eighty-to-eighty-four age category, my peers are few and far between even at the state level. I guess I am outliving the competition.

Every December I write an annual Christmas letter recapping the year. Some highlights from 1998 include my "Sis Is Eighty" birthday party, another Biking Across Kansas event, winning the women's division sixty-and-over Independence Day 8K race, attending the New Mexico State Senior Olympics where I set records in the women's eighty-and-over category, and attending the first ever reunion of my college's Drum and Bugle Corp, of which I was a member from 1936 to 1940. I hadn't seen these people in over fifty years. It was quite a homecoming.

When I finish a race there is usually a gaggle of people who stay to cheer for me. Everyone wants to talk to the old lady. They want to know how old I am and how long I've been doing this. They ask me for advice, as if I am the Ann Landers of aging. I tell them it is never too late to start. Whatever you can do now is your start. By the time you reach fifty or sixty and feel like slowing down, you have to force yourself to move. Sure it's tough. Sometimes it hurts. Sure it's easier to let other people do things for you while you sit on the couch. But if you can't get moving at sixty, you'll lose it forever. My own mother was in a nursing home at this age. She didn't move enough. When I finish a six-mile race I'm tired and dragging but happy I did it. Maybe I come in last, but that's not the point. I see other women my age or even younger who have fallen into the "sit down and do it for me" mode and you just can't do that. I get up at 4:15 in the morning to get in my mile run and then do some calisthenics. Of course I feel like staying in bed next to Bob, who is still sleeping soundly. But I make myself do it.

Out of all the thousands of awards I have earned, I am most proud of the New Mexico Golden Athlete Award, which I received in 1998. The selection is based on athletic ability, community service, and efforts to further senior programs. I had to write a brief statement on my contributions for enhancing the quality of life of seniors and I often reflect on that and quote from it when I give lectures. I just tell seniors to *keep moving!* It is the most important way of enhancing the quality of their lives. Don't follow the time-worn advice given most to seniors, which is to slow down. Never slow down.

THE SWIMMING STOIC

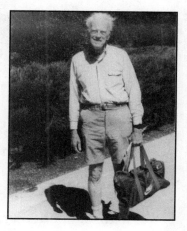

JOHN WOODS

Date of birth: 2-6-18

Residence:
North Harpswell, Maine

**"When a man has said, "I have lived," every morning
he arises, he receives a bonus." —Cicero**

*John Woods has lived a full life. A navy pilot in World War II, and
a commerical pilot afterwards, he retired to a fruit farm in Costa
Rice. Ten years later he retired again to a house and small boat in
Maine. Throughout his life, running and swimming have given him
exercise and pleasure. But it wasn't until his eighties that the concept
of age-group athletics opened his eyes to just how much exercise
helps delay the aging process. John still chops and stacks his own
woodpile in anticipation of those long Maine winters and keeps
busy with swimming, running, and holding his own with the students at the Bowdoin College pool. Never one to feel his age, he
enjoys the fact that he is the youngest swimmer on his relay team.*

I injured my knee the other day getting out of the pool after
my workout. Sitting on the deck, I bent my knee to stand but
pulled it a little too sharply and heard a popping sound followed by instant pain. A trip to the orthopedic surgeon confirmed the need for arthroscopic surgery to clean out some

cartilage damage. Afterwards, the doctor commented on how lucky I was to have the bone structure of a forty-year-old man. It was a great compliment considering that I am eighty-one.

Although born in New York City, I never adjusted to city life; it was too confining. Both my parents had New England roots so maybe that's where my love for the country and a need for space came from. Visits to my grandmother were the best part of early childhood. For one, I adored her, and the visits got me out of the city. The other reason was the 3,000 acres with a pond that Grandmother lived on. I messed around quite a bit there, occasionally getting into trouble. I think I burned down her tool shed among other horrible things kids do. Little boys and matches are not a good mix. And then there were the boating expeditions on the reservoir by her house with the NO SWIMMING sign posted. Many times that darn boat managed to overturn and dump us in the water so we would have to swim a bit.

A severe case of asthma plagued me as a child. What was needed was a change of climate, so at the age of seven I found myself at boarding school in Arizona. Eventually the condition cleared up, as a result of the drier climate and just growing out of it. During those years participation in endurance sports was limited and I was no good at hand-eye coordination, so sports such as baseball or basketball were not the answer. However, after the asthma cleared up I participated in crew and soccer. In high school I played football, not because I wanted to but due to the peer pressure of not wanting to be labeled a sissy. Back then, and I fear perhaps still now, it was declared that people who didn't play football were sissies. My short football career was spent shining the bench with my uniform.

After graduating from Harvard in 1940, I joined the navy pilot training program, as we all knew the war was coming. I was a navy pilot for almost eight years, flying seventy-two combat missions in the Pacific in a twin-engine bomber. It was an exciting time on the cutting edge of the war effort. It was a tremendous privilege to be part of this with thousands of people working in factories and otherwise supporting us. We flew air cover for some of the bloodiest battles in the Pacific. Our planes were small and fast, and luckily we were always able to outrun the Japanese. After the war I tried a few industry jobs but went back to flying and became a pilot for American Airlines. It was a wonderful job and a wonderful way to get back to the exhilaration of flying. Basically, flying was all I knew how to do, so it made sense to stay in the field. With a schedule of two days on and three days off and great pay, it afforded me the opportunity to have the lifestyle I wanted, living in rural Connecticut.

After ten years with American Airlines I wanted to see if I could use my brain as well as my hands so I quit the airlines and was elected to the Connecticut General Assembly. Although I was using my brain, the pay was not so great, so I moved to Washington, D.C., for an aviation position. Along the way, probably at age forty, I picked up jogging to stay in shape. I wasn't killing myself; just moved along adequately enough. However, while in Washington I upgraded from a jogger to a serious runner. One of the reasons I took running more seriously was to get in better shape. I didn't like my physical condition. At six foot one with a tall frame, my weight could have been somewhat leaner. Through running, I was able to maintain an average weight of 150, at one point dropping to 146. Over time, serious running led to serious

training, which led to competition. More and more bitten by
the bug, I started traveling to events. The other part of running that captured me was the people. I met so many lovely
people through the various running clubs and attending the
competitions, thus making a lot of friends throughout the
years. Of course I would be remiss not to mention another
reason for the running: ego and vanity. Don't let anyone tell
you this doesn't factor into the equation.

For thirty years my average weekly mileage was fifty, top-
ping off at eighty. I ran six marathons but didn't really enjoy
them. One has to invest so much time in the training and
then afterward it takes too much time to recover. I remember
running my one and only Boston Marathon, which is like
running through a circus. When departing Boston at the air-
port, when they wheeled the stairs up to the door of the plane
(remember, this is quite a while back). I had to climb the
stairs backwards while the stewardess roared with laughter.
Although I wasn't crazy about the marathon, it was my best
distance. At sixty-one years of age, I ran the Marine Corps
Marathon in three hours and twenty-four minutes. That was
my best time ever. During my stay in the Washington area, I
usually placed number one in my age group at the races. This
is attributable to having good endurance—and of course running ten miles a day didn't hurt. I often get asked why I ran
so much and what I got out of it. Was it for health reasons, for
ego? To answer that, I must tell you a story that takes place in
Rome, Italy, the site of the World Games when I was sixty-
five. A bunch of us were sitting around on the dusty and dirty
floor of the former registration and central meeting place for
the games. The officials had decided to give third place
medals down through eighth place. It took hours for them to

untangle the paper trail that led to the list of final names, and while we sat there waiting, one man got up and said, "Why are we all here waiting? Yes, running is good for us. Yes, running has wonderful health benefits and we enjoy it. So knowing that, why are we all sitting around on a dusty floor waiting for a five-cent piece of tin to hang around our necks?" That's where the ego and vanity come into the picture, as well as self-esteem. A few pieces of tin can attest to the fact that we are athletes. With these pieces of tin we can absorb crushing blows to the ego more easily than if we don't have any other way to tell ourselves we are as good as we'd like to think of ourselves as being.

At age sixty-two, I'd had enough of bureaucracy and said good-bye to Washington and retired to Costa Rica. I messed around a bit, managed a fruit farm, ran every day, and with sufficient knowledge of Spanish got myself involved in the community. I played my guitar, depending on the definition of the word *play*, which I don't do all that well, and attended the symphony and generally loved my life down there. My daughters would come down to visit and we led quite a nice life. I stayed for ten years and then moved to Maine. When I returned to the States, my running was beginning to hurt the bottom of one foot. It got bad enough to visit a doctor—in fact many doctors, none of whom could diagnose the problem. Finally, the umpteenth doctor was knowledgeable enough to find the cause. He confirmed that my metatarsal arches were inflamed. After all the years of pounding, my natural cushion and shock absorber quit and I was forced to retire the running shoes. However, I didn't sit down for long.

Swimming was the replacement for running. I was always a recreational swimmer, but I was never coached or trained properly. With competitive swimming, I really came into my own in the pool, actually turning out to be a better swimmer than runner. In the beginning of my training I attended seminars and listened to coaches about form and fitness and routines, but I found that the more I listened, the more the experts disagreed. I started to ask my buddies for advice, and that's how I learned. My endurance in the pool allowed me to go longer distances without running out of energy. In 1998 I won two gold medals and a silver medal at the nationals for the eighty-to-eighty-four age group. I did better in 1997, but the eighties division was peaceful then. Now it's a busy lane. There were sixteen competitors in one event alone. At masters events you can't tell who won a heat and who came in last due to the age divisions. In fact, the person who finishes last often gets more applause than the winner.

The idea of age-group athletics is the best thing that happened to delaying the aging process. No one is discriminated against by his or her age or ability. No one is ever left out. There are many people who would never think to pick up a sport or try a new activity—especially at a senior age—for fear of failure or, worse, fear of being laughed at. With age-group athletics, all of that is water under the bridge. A sixty-year old is not going to be made to look foolish by a twenty-year-old. It brings together people who belong together. The Road Runners Club of America started a program called, RFYL, which stands for "Run for Your Life." It was purposely created to reach people who hardly thought of exercise before, who didn't think they could do it. They were given the track for a two-mile run. It was a very successful endeavor. Those who were encouraged to try felt good about their abilities. I do remember once a more experienced runner entered the meet and was yelling at others to get out of his way. We had to ask him to stop. He didn't belong there; he was intimidating the very people we were trying to convert.

I try to exercise every day, and vary my routine. If I skip a day of swimming, I'll work out with free weights or run. And after years of laying off running, my foot healed itself and now I run seven miles a week and enter about three races a year. I'm not as fast as I was, plugging away at a ten-minute pace, but I'm out there and that's what's important. I also write a newsletter for the Maine Masters Swim Club and try to keep my house and property in some semblance of order. And as soon as the first frost hits the air, which happens early up here, I start loading up on the firewood and cart it to the house. I did five barrelfuls this morning. I also enjoy my little boat, which I've cruised all over for fourteen years and gives me a great deal of pleasure. And then there's my girlfriend. She lives close by and we're fond of each other, although she can be very demanding at times and likes to order me around. She'll dash into my kitchen, grab me by the hand and insist I take her to the playground. She loves the swings. Most three-year-olds do.

I still try to get down to the family reunions with my daughters in Maryland, but the ten-hour drive is getting a bit taxing for me. My oldest daughter, who lives closer, checks up on me from time to time. And then there's the over-eighty relay swim team, which I put together a few months ago. Our junior man is eighty-one. He had just about given up swimming when I called him. It made his day to know that we needed him. All his motivation came back. The team is then rounded out with two eighty-three-year olds. This could probably be the first eighty-and-over relay team in Maine.

Our target is the Master National Swimming Championships.

I've been very lucky to always have friends of all ages. It is important to all age groups to intermingle as much as possible and share the various learning that is going on at all levels. I don't get to see my grandchildren as often as I'd like, but through my neighbor's daughter—my girlfriend—I know how busy and active they can be. I've been swimming at the Bowdoin College pool for many years now, becoming friendly with the students on the swim team, even officiating at some of their meets.

I'd like to tell you that I jump out of bed every morning bursting with energy to start the day, but I kind of like being lazy in the morning. There are so many things I have to get done, there is need to think about them, reflect on what to do first. But then I get around to putting one foot in front of the other and look forward to another day.

A UNIVERSAL MAN

HAROLD ZINKIN

Date of birth: 5-11-22

Residence: Fresno, California

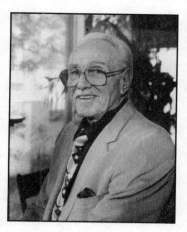

"I am long on ideas, but short on time. I expect to live to be only about a hundred." —Thomas Edison

Zinkin may not be a recognizable name, but people who work out at gyms and health clubs are more familiar with Harold then they realize. He grew up with the original fitness crowd back in the 1930s on Muscle Beach in Santa Monica, California. After the war, Harold continued his healthy habits and strength training, dedicating his life to exercise and fitness. An outgrowth of this dedication was inventing the Universal Gym equipment used in health clubs today all over the world. A depression-era kid who didn't know where his next meal was coming from, at seventy-seven Harold is president of an international corporation that supplies cardiovascular fitness equipment to homes and businesses. A survivor of a double-bypass heart operation, Harold still gets in his daily workout and feels that his exercise routine is the key ingredient in keeping him fit and alive.

Growing up during the depression era was tough on most everyone. My father earned fifteen dollars a week. There was no time for kids to have fun—we were too busy working jobs after school or standing on food lines for a loaf of bread that would be dinner for the week. I wanted to play like other ordinary kids but spent my spare time mopping floors for extra money. My main interest in life, besides work, was fitness. Even back in elementary school, I was fascinated by fitness and bodybuilding. And of course there was a female in the picture, a young blonde who was part of a traveling gymnast show. She couldn't have been more than ten years old, my contemporary, and I'd watch her tumble in wonderful vivid outfits of pink and purple. We got to be friends and her mother sewed my name on her outfits.

As a teenager I worked in a bowling alley for twenty-five cents an hour setting up the pins. I had to adjust them quickly, hoping to hell the guy at the other end wasn't drunk and the big black ball wouldn't come crashing down at me. I could handle the job because I was very physical and strong. Always was. The older guys liked to show me off because I could beat anyone. Although money was tight, I'd scrape my nickels and dimes together to buy a magazine dedicated to bodybuilding and fitness called *Physical Culture*, read it end to end, then share it with my friends. By sixteen I was participating in tumbling and strength exercises at the famous Muscle Beach in Santa Monica, the birthplace of the physical fitness boom in the twentieth century. Thousands came to watch the activities. To me this was sheer excitement, what I must have been waiting for. A sports boom was taking hold in our country, sparked by Jesse Owens at the 1936 Olympics in Germany. Hitler had made big overtures that Aryan supremacy would conquer the sports arena, and there was Jesse with four gold medals in track. The world will never forget when Hitler refused to meet with him. Owens was great and he helped bring the world of fitness nearer to me.

I've never pursued anything else more vigorously in my life. My buddies and I helped prove to the world that through exercise and proper diet you could have the type of body you want. We worked hard, but it was fun and rewarding. That's a key ingredient. If it's not rewarding, who's going to do it? The guys and girls I worked out with at Muscle Beach ruled the fitness world: Jack LaLanne, Vic and Armand Tanny, Joe Gold. In fact it was my friend Vic Tanny who entered me into the first Mr. California contest without my knowing it in 1941. At nineteen I was the youngest entrant and didn't think I had a chance. The sound of the applause when they announced I had won still rings in my ears today.

Some folks referred to us as muscleheads and didn't understand what we were all about. We were different, I'll grant you that—but not freaks. Just healthier and enjoyed life a great deal more than most. Some of us were even vegetarians, almost unheard of back then. But it's interesting that none of us ended our careers at Muscle Beach. Just the contrary. We all took what we loved and brought it to the masses for their education and benefit. It's not too much of a stretch to say we influenced the way the world looked at fitness. We evolved from a group having fun with our routines to staging shows and giving free instruction. People came to admire the strong healthy bodies they saw and left wondering if they could do the same. It was pure and they saw that. Then Joe Weider started his muscle magazine, the younger kids started participating and the evolution continued. Even Roy Rogers occasionally got into the act. And after the war, servicemen joined us at Muscle Beach. Many had never worked out before the service and wanted to continue and improve upon the minimal training they received in wartime. Arnold Schwarzenegger came to the beach to work out when he came to the United States.

When I got the idea to open up a fitness gym in 1948 with my partner Bruce Conner, I announced the opening and invited doctors to send us their patients who needed to lose or gain weight or just get in shape. When our first clients started to arrive, they'd tell us the only instructions received from the doctor, were to get in shape. That did not present a problem to me, as during World War II I enlisted to fight but instead was sent to physical instructors' and rehabilitation schools. I ended up at Long Beach Naval Hospital helping to heal the injured servicemen. My background in physical therapy was put to use on my new clients. At Bruce's and my gym, everyone who walked in the door had to first fill in a questionnaire. They were asked to list any illnesses, their purpose in coming to the gym, if they were referred by a doctor or came on their own accord, and any joint restrictions. The last one was for my staff so they wouldn't unknowingly hurt a client during a workout. That card is still used in many gyms. The basic routine consisted of the following: warm-up stretches, endurance exercises for the cardiovascular system and strength exercises. Don't let the term *strength exercise* fool you. Gravity alone is a resistive exercise. Sometimes we'd use one-pound weights, sometimes no weights. A set of power walks up and down a flight of stairs will work anyone over. All my instructors were personal trainers and you didn't have to hire them separately at extra cost. That was their job. They didn't stand around idle. I will tell you from my heart that all my life's work in the gyms was never for money. I did it to help others and spread the word about the benefits of fitness.

Over the years there's been a growing trend of older people joining gyms, which is wonderful. There's been a lot of positive changes in the industry over the years, and one of the most influential changes is the exercise shows on television. They are reaching and motivating millions of people. Some are actually borderline fantastic and it's great for older people who can't or won't get out to a gym. Then again, beware of the charlatans. You can spot them by what they promise in their ads. No one is going to lose ten pounds by doing two weeks of sit-ups. Stay away from anyone guaranteeing you can take an inch off your waist and lose ten pounds in a week or two. It's almost impossible to do healthfully. The standard measure of loss for waist reduction for most body types is approximately one inch for five pounds lost. This goes along with following careful nutritional guidelines along with exercise, and most likely will take up to a month instead of two weeks. And you don't need to buy equipment or costly supplements either.

There are no miracles. It all boils down to the amount of energy you are willing to put into the program. There is no exercise on this earth where you can lie down, sleep, wake up and lose weight. Doesn't happen that way. You have to tax yourself a little bit each day, show some sensible effort, don't overdo it, and eventually your fitness will improve. It's really very basic, no different than tending a garden. If you progressively work with a hoe or rake, over time you will develop a protective covering, a callus, on your hands—as opposed to a blister, which is an irritation. The callus will harden and your skin will become tough. If you progressively work your cardiovascular system, your heart, like your skin, becomes stronger. Through exercise, the body will respond and build resistance. Tax your body—get stronger and healthier. Be tough with yourself, as well as sensible. Medical science has assured us a stronger, longer vigorous life if we do. But people are not always sensible. The average American now eats about 160 calories more each day than back in the 1970s. That wouldn't be a problem if the extra weight was being worked off with exercise, but unfortunately just the opposite is true. When it comes to physical activity, Americans are doing less. More calories, less activity. It doesn't take a genius to figure the outcome. According to a recent Harvard health publication, more than half of American adults are considered moderately overweight and almost a quarter are significantly overweight. The easiest way to cut down on daily calories is to look at serving suggestions. The suggested serving size for a bowl of cereal is typically two-thirds of a cup but the average bowl of cereal we eat is three to four times larger. Don't underestimate your calorie intake. Here's a simple tip: Learn to judge more accurately just how much you are indeed eating.

While developing routines for use at the gyms, I saw a need for new equipment. There wasn't any one piece that hit all the body parts and was simple to use. I worked on prototypes of equipment at a local machine shop, looking for a way to combine the stacks of weights and barbells into one machine. Between 1957 and 1960 I applied for and received from the U.S. Patent Office most of the patents necessary to create the revolutionary Universal Gym Machine. We started off selling one a month, then one a week, and then one an hour. The rest is history. Eventually I registered six U.S. patents related to the Universal Gym Machine, which revolutionized the industry. Thirty years after the first machine rolled off the assembly line,I received a call from my high school football coach. Back then I went against his rule that no one works out with weights. He said it'd only make us slow and muscle-bound. Then he'd add, "Only that crazy Zinkin can use them, because he's different." Thirty years later and now a principal of another high school, he called me personally to order a Universal Machine for his school. It was quite a moment for us both.

The older you get, the more important it is to exercise. When you are young, every day is usually filled with running around, doing errands, bending, moving, and being flexible. We tend to stop doing those things as we age and get sedentary. The blood circulation slows down and the body starts to deteriorate faster. If an older person isn't fit then everyday chores, even such as food shopping and handling become a drudgery or, worse, impossible. How are you going to lift the bags, carry them into the house, and lift your arms to put the food away on a top shelf if you've lost most of your strength and bone mass? Cardiovascular training is probably the most important thing for long life—that and nutrition. Participation in regular physical activity is the one change that can have the greatest impact on health and longevity. Just for basic survival, you should be in shape. An inactive body is a deteriorating body. The earlier you poop out on exercise, the harder your remaining years will be. If I don't live another minute, I'll die happy knowing I lived seventy-seven active, full years.

As happy as I was with my life at the time, I was also extremely busy. Always a businessman, my one gym grew into thirty fitness centers and the Universal Gym Machine grew into one of the largest fitness companies in the world.

My fingers also worked their way into real estate development in Fresno. Eventually tension and stress took their toll in the way of double-bypass heart surgery when I was sixty-four. Luckily, it was only a wake-up call and not the final note. I left the hospital after a relatively short stay due to my high level of fitness. The doctor said if I can walk half a mile I can go home, and that was a piece of cake. Exercise is a major ingredient in keeping you alive. Every day my workout program consists of a two-hour cardiovascular workout, walking two or three miles, followed by a thirty-minute resistive training routine using my Universal Machine and free weights. I don't do heavy resistance anymore, trying to accomplish everything in ten to twelve repetitions. Instead I'll do twenty to thirty repetitions with lighter weights. It's never boring, as the time is used to work on my projects, return phone calls, or catch up on the news. I have ten telephones within easy access so no one trying to reach me ever feels left out or cut short. My exercise creed is simple: "If you don't miss one workout, you won't miss two."

My experience at Muscle Beach made a profound difference in my life. It taught me to think about fitness— to think about possibilities rather than impossibilities, about my own strengths that went beyond my muscles. I wouldn't have wanted to live life any other way. That and being close with my family, seeing my grandsons perform perfect handstands, help get me out of bed in the morning.

SEPARATING THE MEDICAL MYTHS FROM THE FACTS ABOUT AGING

AN INTERVIEW WITH DR. WALTER BORTZ

**"If you look into the eyes of the young you see flame.
If you look into the eyes of the old you see light."
—Victor Hugo**

Dr. Walter Bortz is one of America's most respected and acclaimed authorities on aging. The former president of the American Geriatrics Society, he cochaired the American Medical Association Task Force on Aging. Presently a clinical associate professor at Stanford University Medical School, he also has his own practice that specializes in elders. Dr. Bortz is also a distance runner, and veteran of many marathons and an active member of the Fifty-Plus Fitness Association. He is also the author of We Live Too Short and Die Too Long *and* Dare to Be 100. *The following interview represents some of his views on the aging process.*

THE GIFT OF FOUND TIME

Birth certificates don't come with expiration dates stamped on them." says Dr. Bortz. "They are an open-ended ticket to a long and healthy life. However, some people cut that life short, either mentally or physically, when they start to age. What exactly is aging? Is it a disease, a process, a behavior, a symptom? It lacks a conceptual framework. It is not an exaggeration to assert that everything we have been taught about aging has been wrong. No one dies of old age. Dr. Robert Butler, first director of the National Institute on Aging, has said, 'We have not found any biological reason not to live to 110.' For conditions of old people not to be due to the passage of time gives hope that counterstrategies can be derived to prevent or reverse at least a major part of them."

FACTS VERSUS MYTHS

Throughout history humans have been mistaking disease for the hallmarks of aging. Conditions as diverse as tuberculosis, hardening of the arteries, and Alzheimer's disease have in the past been conceded by practitioners to be due to aging. The error in this miscategorization is now clear. By putting the correct label, *disease*, on arteriosclerosis, fate is replaced by the prevention or treatment. People don't die of a heart attack, they succumb to a lifelong habit of neglect and disuse. Old people don't just get Alzheimer's disease. Heart attacks, strokes, arthritis, emphysema, and cirrhosis are common examples of medical conditions due to dissonance, or imbalance. Dr. Bortz is very clear on distinguishing a disease that is preventable and curable from conditions over which the person afflicted has little or no control, such as genetic diseases like sickle-cell anemia. Other conditions such as injuries, infections and malignancies, which used to be a death seal, are preventable and sometimes curable thanks to years of research funding and studies. Unfortunately more of these diseases, such as Alzheimer's, knock at the door every day. Then there is the group that Dr. Bortz labels *dissonance condi-*

tions. "These conditions are the direct result of the inappropriate relationship of the person with his or her environment. They take years to develop, but once encountered do not lend themselves easily to cure. Dissonance comes in two forms of imbalance to the system: too much, i.e. stress, or too little, i.e. disuse." Here are a few examples of dissonance conditions.

HEART DISEASE

Dr. Bortz describes the number one killer in our country as not really a heart problem but rather an artery problem. "A heart attack is hardening of the arteries or arteriosclerosis—blocked arteries. A forty-year-old with bad pipes can be old; an eighty-year-old with clean pipes can be young. It has been estimated that if arteriosclerosis were eliminated, a person sixty-five years of age could accrue from ten to sixteen years of additional life. Diet and exercise can eliminate the cause of a heart attack. Nearly 800,000 Americans die each year in the confusion we call heart disease."

CANCER

Does taking a walk help prevent cancer? There is increasing evidence that cancer is not just a random event—that it really has a strong relationship to how we live our lives.

According to Bortz, "More and more researchers are finding that physical fitness helps us prevent cancer. No one suggests that being fit eliminates the risk of cancer altogether, but numerous studies strikingly illustrate lower rates of the disease in people who exercise. Some forms of cancer seem particularly responsive to an active lifestyle, colon cancer among them. Other cancers such as lung cancer are also low in fit persons, but this is felt to be due to the fact that few fit people smoke."

OSTEOPOROSIS

Osteo—meaning bone—and *porosis*—meaning porous—is a disease that's due to the gradual decline from disuse of muscle mass. Ninety percent of women over seventy-five have osteoporosis and more than eighteen million people have low bone mass. However, this disease is both preventable and treatable; it doesn't just happen. There is a basic law of bone structure, called Wolff's Law, which asserts that "the robusticity of any bone is in direct proportion to the physical stresses applied to it." Dr. Bortz sums up the law this way, "Use it or lose it." A group of French researchers discovered that thirty-six weeks in bed can provoke the same amount of calcium loss from bones as seen in ten years of aging. Weight-bearing activities have proven to be a successful step in reducing the risks of osteoporosis.

ALZHEIMER'S DISEASE

Alzheimer's is a disease, not a condition of the aging process. It is the fourth leading cause of death for people over age sixty-five, yet the research budget for AD remains trivial. The predominant symptom is loss of memory—generally recent memory—but there is no definitive test for Alzheimer's. Bortz, who has testified on Alzheimer's before a committee of the House of Representatives, says, "In my view, the major tragedy of Alzheimer's is not with those with the disease or their grieving families, but with the rest of us who mistakenly take this forlorn vision to reflect the true face of aging. Alzheimer's disease is not aging. Most people, most old people, never get it."

FRAILTY

Frailty is not congruous with aging. It is a predisposition to failure found even in young people, mostly due to malnutrition. It is the opposite of vitality. Aging does contribute to frailty—a ninety-year-old is not the same as a twenty-year-old, but even a ninety-year-old can recapture lost vigor with an exercise program. Again, Dr. Bortz goes back to his theory of disuse when speaking about frailty. "Frailty results from disuse more than it does from aging. Frailty is not aging, and it is reversible. But left unattended, the progressive development of frailty leads to increased susceptibility to other conditions. At thirty we can withstand a fractured hip easily; at ninety a fractured hip can be fatal to a person with frail conditions. A critical lesson learned from frailty is that the losses to time, while real, are inconsequential when compared to the losses due to disuse. A fit seventy-year-old has lost the same amount of vitality as an unfit person many years younger. Fitness is a thirty-to forty-year age offset. Fitness for a young person is an option; but for the elder person an imperative."

SUCCESSFUL AGING

The terms *successful* and *usual* in connection with aging are used universally to denote the two trajectories of aging people. Usual aging is the standard, commonplace variety.

Successful aging represents the theoretical ideal. There are changes due to aging that are real, measurable, and significant. But when contrasted to the changes due to disuse, they are unimportant to overall function. Usual aging is now quantified as a 2 percent decrement per year of overall function, whereas the successful aging rate is only 0.5 percent per year. Bortz knows firsthand the reality of the application of these percentages. "As a long-distance runner, I identify easily that I am slower than I was thirty years ago. But turn me loose against an unfit thirty-year-old and I will leave him or her panting in my wake. Fitness compensates, even overcompensates, for age loss. Aging well requires stamina and effort. You must be sound of body, mind, and social environment if you are to live and age ideally."

STEPPING-STONES TO A LONG LIFE

Exercise plays a key role in every aspect of Dr. Bortz's program regarding successful aging. And using himself as a role model, he knows it isn't easy. That first step toward an exercise program is the hardest and most important. Good intentions remain only good intentions until you follow them with action. According to a report issued by the U.S. surgeon general, only 15 percent of Americans now engage in moderate physical activity like brisk walking, swimming, cycling, dancing or doing yardwork for at least thirty minutes at a time, five or more times a week. And only 23 percent engage in vigorous physical activity like jogging, lap swimming, and racket sports for twenty or more minutes at a time three or more days a week. Bortz likes to put a spin on the list of excuses he hears about not starting an exercise program. "The thought

'I'm too old to exercise' should be translated into 'I'm too old not to exercise.' Physical exercise exerts beneficial effects on virtually every bodily function: body weight, blood pressure, HDL cholesterol (the good kind), blood clotting, respiratory function, sexual capacity, glucose tolerance, immunology capacity, and behavioral characteristics such as mood, cognition and memory." Exercise has even more positive side effects. Recent studies have found that exercise is good for the brain. During any form of exertion, blood is shifted from the unessential parts of the body—such as the intestine and kidneys—to the arms and legs, where the work is going on. The brain, however, is spared this diversion. It continues to receive its pint and a half of blood every minute. Exercise prompts the release of adrenaline, a very potent brain stimulant. We are more alert when adrenaline is present, so in effect, exercise increases the IQ. It is reported that smart people exercise more. Bortz poses the question, "Do they exercise because they are smart, or are they smart because they exercise?" A new study suggests that taking an invigorating walk gives the brains of people sixty to seventy-five years old a good workout, sharpening both memory and judgment. Exercise is also a mood enhancer. Movement is good for you. Psychologists and psychiatrists have embraced the notion that physical exercise is an important form of therapy for depressed people. "One of the various effects of adrenaline is to act as a stimulus for the release of endorphins in the brain. Endorphins are chemicals that nature has created to make us pain insensitive. Together, adrenaline and endorphins are uppers, nature's way of treating depression through exercise."

LESSONS FROM OUR ELDERS

Centenarians are the most rapidly growing segment of the American population. With regard to health, they rate the importance of mobility as being tightly linked to survival. Ninety-one percent of male centenarians can walk, as well as 85 percent of women. Next to working, walking is considered the best old-age prescription. Belle Boone writes in *Centenarians: The New Generation*, "Nothing is more detrimental to the health and happiness of very old people than to deny them the privilege of walking." In general, centenarians wisely disregard advice to take it easy.

EXERCISE ADVICE

Dr. Bortz gives us his own views regarding an exercise program, no matter what sport you choose.

WHAT TYPE OF EXERCISE?

Cardiovascular conditioning—anything that works the heart, lungs, blood vessels, blood cells, muscles, tendons, and bones to their highest working efficiency.

HOW MUCH?

Three times a week for half an hour. One session is better than none, two is better than one, and three better than two.

INTENSITY?

We must exert ourselves—stretch ourselves—work ourselves; no bowling, no golf, no gin rummy. The textbooks state that for us to attain fitness we need to exercise at 70 percent of our maximum. One way to measure this is through pulse rate. Like other vital functions, there is a maximum number of times your heart can beat per minute. Exercise raises your heartbeat to its maximum pulse rate. It is linked to age and falls progressively as we age.

Dr. Bortz playfully summarizes his years in the field of health and aging with two words: *Have guts!* All successful older people demonstrate cool courage and a firm competency that accepts—even seeks—challenge. Without challenge, there can be no flow in life, and not to experience and confront challenges would make life a pretty pallid event. You have to have guts to age successfully. Be more than body fit, be whole-person fit—body, mind, spirit, all in harmony, balance, and vitality. This is the ideal. It takes guts. It takes involvement. Just do it."

HOW TO START A RUNNING PROGRAM AT ANY AGE

Contributed by Amby Burfoot, editor of Runner's World *magazine and winner of the 1968 Boston Marathon. Also a recipient of the George Sheehan Award for "outstanding journalistic contributions to the sport of running," and author of* The Principles of Running: Practical Lessons Learned from My First 100,000 Miles.

So you are thinking of becoming a runner. Congratulations! Let me assure you this is probably one of the most pure, fun, easy, painless, and perhaps addictive forms of exercise you can start regardless of age. In fact the older we get, the more important exercise becomes. Some people worry that running is hard on the joints, but there is no scientific evidence to support this, nor do studies prove that it causes or aggravates arthritis. On the contrary, running regularly on soft surfaces with good posture can actually stave off osteoarthritis. And as an added benefit, you burn roughly 120 calories with each mile regardless of speed. Sounds almost too good to be true, but medical and scientific research has proven beyond a doubt that running is one of the healthiest exercises, if not *the* healthiest.

Before I explain how to start a running program, I want to immediately put to rest any concerns or fears you may have about distance and speed. Regarding distance, the length of your run is not as important as the amount of time you exercise. The American College of Sports Medicine suggests that a minimum of ten minutes of exercise at least two days a week will bring physical benefits. Second, don't even think speed. The stopwatch is a cruel master. Remember the fable of the tortoise and hare and you are off to a good start.

We are almost out the door, but not quite. If you haven't been on an exercise program for a while, get a checkup before lacing up the running shoes. Now you are ready.

To Start: Think Minutes Not Miles

—Walk your way into running. For the first week or so walk 90 seconds, run 30 seconds. Repeat 9 more times for a total of 20 minutes. Follow this routine four times a week until you are comfortable. Gradually switch to more running until you can run steadily for 20 minutes.

—If you can run and talk without losing breath, you've reached a comfortable pace. If you can't, slow down until you catch your breath.

—You can't run too slowly. Run comfortably and you will enjoy running for a lifetime.

Moving Forward: The 10 Percent Rule

—The most important principle of running is the 10 percent rule. Never increase your weekly mileage by more than 10 percent over the previous week. This may sound overcautious, but it works. If you follow it, you should avoid injuries due to overtraining.

—Set realistic goals. Aim for the attainable and you won't get discouraged.

Proper Form: It's all in the smile

—Run tall and erect, looking straight ahead or slightly down.

—Keep your shoulders relaxed and your arms swinging comfortably by your sides at hip level.

—Lift your knee just enough to get your leg moving. There's no need to overextend.

—The foot motion is a heel-to-toe push.

Equipment: No Fashion Statement Required

—The one essential ingredient is the right pair of running shoes. Don't choose by color, price, or brand. What's good for your neighbor may not be the right shoe for you. Be picky. Try them on with the socks you will be wearing when you run.

—Be sure to take a brief try-out: Jog around the store before buying. Check the return policy.

—Avoid cotton shirts and socks. Cotton fabric doesn't breathe and will hold sweat and moisture. Buy microfiber materials. They cost slightly more but are well worth it. You'll stay dry and comfortable in all types of weather.

Support Groups: Everyone Needs One Sometime

—Running with a partner can add consistency, enjoyment and moral support to your runs. Don't have one? Contact your local Y and ask about running groups. Scan your newspaper for running columns, advice, lectures or other places where you can seek out other runners. Contact the high school track coach for advice. Join a local running club.

Runners Are Everywhere!

—Finally, remember that exercise makes you feel better and more alive every day. It also gives you more energy, so today's half mile can be next month's mile.

HOW TO START
A SWIMMING PROGRAM
AT ANY AGE

Contributed by Bill Volckening, head coach of the Tualatin Hills Barracudas of Beaverton, Oregon, and editor of the U.S. Masters Swimming organization's Swim *magazine.*

Are you considering becoming a swimmer? Good choice! Swimming is probably one of the healthiest, most enjoyable, challenging, and lowest impact forms of exercise you can do. Regardless of ability level and experience, people of all ages can swim. As we age, it is important to consider adding low impact aerobic exercise to the physical fitness routine. Swimming is the ideal activity for many who can no longer bear the high impact and joint stress of running or jogging. People sometimes worry about swimming's influence on weight loss. Skeptics say it's impossible to lose weight swimming, but it is possible. In fact, combined with a healthy balanced diet, swimming regularly can help people lose weight as easily as other physical activities, such as running. For people who are overweight, swimming is perhaps the best way to exercise, because it alleviates stress on the leg joints. Swimming has the added benefit of providing a total body cardiovascular workout unlike any other.

When starting a swimming routine, as with any other physical fitness activity, make sure to consult with a physician. Start slowly and build up to increase the limits. Remember, speed and distance are not as important as the length of time you swim. According to the American Heart

Association, just thirty to sixty minutes of physical activity three to four days per week can help reduce your risk for heart disease, stroke, and diabetes. A regular physical activity program can also help lower your blood pressure and cholesterol. It is a good idea to monitor your heart rate while swimming. Start by determining a maximum heart rate. In healthy adults with no previous history of heart disease, the maximum heart rate commonly recommended by physicians is the number 220 minus your age. Check your heart rate routinely while exercising by taking your pulse during a ten-second period. Use a clock for better accuracy. After counting the beats for ten seconds, multiply the number by six to get the heart rate.

First Consideration—Equipment

—Swimsuit. Most swimming facilities require swimming suits. Make sure to get one that is comfortable and durable. Several of the swimwear manufacturers offer fuller cut suits for swimmers who prefer the less youthful styles. Some of the newer suits made of polyester will last longer and resist fading.

—Goggles. Protect your eyes and see everything more clearly with goggles. Several manufacturers now make prescription goggles for people who need them. Goggles should be snug yet comfortable. Sometimes it is necessary to keep trying new goggles until you find the right ones.

—Fins. Work your legs and add propulsion to your swimming with fins. There are several kinds to choose from. They should be snug fitting but not too tight. If you can't find the right size, get the slightly larger ones and wear socks with them. Long fins are great for beginners and people who need to develop ankle flexibility. Short fins are an alternative, and they are great for adding speed to your swimming without disproportionately overexerting the leg muscles.

—Pull-buoys. Put some flotation into your swimming by trying a pull-buoy. This piece of equipment is usually made of foam and comes in a variety of shapes and sizes. It is placed between your legs above the knees and allows your lower body to float more while isolating your swimming to the upper body. If your legs tend to sink, or if they're just tired, a pull-buoy can often help.

—Kickboards. If you would like to work your legs exclusively, use a kickboard. This piece of equipment is usually made of foam and comes in a variety of shapes and sizes. It allows your upper body to float while you kick with your legs. If you try a kickboard and find it makes yourshoulders sore, try kicking without it, or try a smaller board with less flotation.

—Hand paddles. If you're looking to work your pull a little more, hand paddles can sometimes help. Hand paddles are usually plastic and are held in place on the hands with short lengths of surgical tubing attached to the paddle. There are other types of paddles that look more like gloves, made of Lycra and rubber. Be careful when considering using hand paddles. They can sometimes put too much stress on the shoulders.

Start Slowly and Build

—Ease into the routine. During the first week try swimming for thirty seconds and resting for thirty seconds. Repeat nine times for a total of ten minutes.

—Now try kicking: Try the same set as above while kicking. Just pick up some fins and go. Kick for thirty seconds and rest for thirty seconds. If you'd like to try a kickboard, most pools will have them available. If your pool doesn't have any, they are inexpensive and last forever.

—Add variety: Try varying the length of your swimming or kicking time in relation to your resting time. When trying to increase the amount of time exercising, start by making the thirty-second swimming time into forty-five seconds while shortening the thirty-second rest period to fifteen seconds. Also try different strokes, such as backstroke, breaststroke, and even butterfly!

—Watch the clock. Pools where competitive teams swim usually have pace clocks installed. Most pace clocks have a sweeping second hand that is usually a bright color. If there is no pace clock, or if you can't see it from the pool, consider purchasing a waterproof watch.

—Build your routine. Start with two or three days a week, and build your routine to include more days if you are comfortable. Make sure to take enough rest to catch your breath between repeats. If thirty seconds of rest is not enough between swims, adjust your rest interval.

—You can't swim too slowly. Swim comfortably and you will enjoy it for a lifetime. Don't worry about how fast other swimmers are, unless you are preparing to enter a lane with other swimmers. Be honest with yourself about the pace you are able to maintain. If you are not a fast swimmer, do not enter a lane with fast swimmers.

Moving Ahead

—Consider the 10 percent rule that runners often use. Avoid increasing your weekly distance by more than 10 percent over the previous week. This may sound overcautious, but it works. If you follow it, you should avoid injuries due to overtraining.

—Set realistic goals. Aim for the attainable and you won't get discouraged. There are many ways to set goals in swimming. It could be as simple as learning to do the stroke better or counting your laps. The most important thing is to have fun with it.

—Technique. Swimming is far more technical than most other activities. Even the best swimmers continue to improve by refining their technique. It is often beneficial to have an instructor or a coach look at you while you swim. People who teach swimming often have suggestions about how to make your swimming more efficient and more enjoyable.

—Lane etiquette. Make sure you know the pool's rules about how to share a lane with other swimmers. When three or more swimmers are sharing a lane, do circle-swimming. Go up on one side of the lane and return on the other. If you are not sure about it, ask the lifeguard, who is there to assist. Watching the traffic patterns is always a good idea before entering a lane with other swimmers.

—Swimming with a partner or a group can help you stay motivated. If you're looking for a partner or a group, go to your local pool and ask about masters swimming groups. Resources are available through U.S. Masters Swimming, which has a website (www.usms.org). Joining a local Masters team is a great way to learn and add camaraderie to your fitness routine. You do not have to go to the competitions to enjoy Masters swimming, but swim meets for seniors can be great fun, too! Swimming is the most popular fitness activity for all ages.

Remember, the cardiovascular benefits of swimming make you feel great. It is exhausting and energizing all at once, and you can do it your entire life.

HOW TO CHOOSE A HEALTH AND SPORTS CLUB

Contributed by Joe Gold, founder of Gold's Gym and World Gym.

As the benefits of exercise become better known, more people of all ages are jumping on the exercise bandwagon and that includes joining health clubs. According to the U.S. surgeon general, "People of all ages should include a minimum of thirty minutes of physical activity of moderate intensity on most, if not all, days of the week. Cardio-respiratory endurance activity should be supplemented with strength-developing exercises at least twice per week for adults, in order to improve musculoskeletal health, maintain independence in performing the activities of daily life, and reduce the risk of falling." I encourage people at all ages and all levels to work out and make it a routine for life.

If you are exercising for the first time, it is suggested that you get a physician's approval before starting any program. After that, follow these basic guidelines for selecting a gym and go out there and enjoy yourself. You'll be doing yourself a favor for a better, and productive and rewarding life.

To Start: Reasons Why People Join Health Clubs

—To exercise regularly in a motivating environment and receive guidance from a built-in support staff of qualified fitness professionals.

—To work out on a variety of user-friendly cardiovascular

and resistance equipment.

—To exercise in a safe environment where CPR, emergency response, and other safeguards are available.

—To have a place to exercise when it is too hot, too cold or hazardous outdoor weather conditions prevail.

—To make new friends of all ages and take advantage of club activities.

How to Find a Reputable Club

—Ask around among friends and family members who belong to a health club and check out their recommendations.

—Check out a local Y for referrals or go through the local newspapers for advertisements of health clubs.

—Call the International Health, Racquet, and Sportsclub Association, the trade group for health clubs, for a listing of member club in your area. (1-800-766-1278).

Ask The Right Questions

—Make sure the club you're looking at is convenient to your home or place of work.

—Visit the facility during the hours you plan to use it and take note of the number of people. Is it too crowded? Is there a wait for the equipment?

—Take a tour of all the rooms at the club: the exercise rooms, changing facilities, showers, lockers, and so on. Is it clean and well maintained?

—Is the equipment state of the art? Is there enough variety of equipment?

—Is the staff available and on the floor, accessible at all times for information and assistance?

—Check to see that there are adequate parking spaces available so that parking your car doesn't become an aerobic exercise.

Senior Citizens: Look for the Following Special Needs

—Make sure the club has a program specific to your age and that the staff is accustomed to working with the senior segment. Are they knowledgeable regarding special medical considerations?

—Check to see that the pound increments of the weights include small intervals such as 3, 5, 8, 10, and 12—and that they don't jump from 5 to 10 to 15.

—Make sure the staff will interact with your doctor if you are on a special program.

Taking the Step Toward Membership

—Ask if they give discounts to seniors or if there is any kind of special membership for coming at off-peak hours.

—Examine the contract carefully. Make sure you understand all the arrangements and that everything agreed to is spelled out in the contract.

—Understand the length of the contract term. Did you sign up for a month, a year, multiyear? Be aware that lifetime memberships are illegal in most states.

—Ask about a cancellation clause and any obligations and

responsibilities you may have if you need to get out of the contract.

—Find out what will happen to the contract if the club goes out of business or sells to a third party.

—Check out the club's profile with the Better Business Bureau to see if any complaints have been filed against it.

Now all you need is the discipline, drive, and determination to go to the club and use it!

ORGANIZATIONS FOR SENIOR ATHLETICS AND ACTIVITIES

Elderhostel
75 Federal Street
Boston, MA 02110
(617) 426-7788

Elder Treks
597 Markham Street
Toronto, Ontario, Canada M6G 2L7
(800) 741-7956

Fifty-Plus Fitness Association
P.O. Box D
Stanford, CA 94309
(415) 323-6160
website: www.50plus.org
e-mail: fitness@ix.netcom.com.

Huntsman World Senior Games
82 West 700 South
St. George, UT 84770
1-800-562-1268
hwsg@infowest.com

U.S. Masters Swimming, Inc.
2 Peter Avenue
Rutland, MA 01543
(508) 886-6631
Fax: (508) 886-6265
www.usms.org

U.S. National Senior Sports Organization
14323 South Outer Forty Road, Suite N300
Chesterfield, MO 63017
(314) 878-4900

Senior Ventures Network, Sikiyou Center
South Oregon State College
Ashland, OR 97520
(800) 257-0577
www.thirdage.com

Real Age: What's Your Real Age? Website
www.realage.com

LESSONS LEARNED

The people in this book are not superstars, super seniors or professional athletes. They are retirees, grandparents, widows, employed personnel, and happily married couples. They could be your neighbors or your parents. If they are "gifted," it is in their attitude toward life. It has been proven that a healthy attitude greatly extends an individual's life span. The common denominator they all share is facing each day with a renewed zest for what lies ahead. And for them, each day is filled with a task list that usually doesn't get completed. They all lead active lives that include goals, responsibilities, families, friends, and exercise.

The number one contributor to leading a successful senior life is work. A recent survey of older Americans found that 40 percent are working for pay in retirement, while an equal percentage do volunteer work. Older people are demanding a more vital and participatory role in life, and are getting it one way or another. Sixty-five percent of retirees view their new found time as a way to begin a new chapter in life by being active and involved. Certainly this population of aging baby boomers will not settle for the sedentary life of retirement that most of their parents did. Retirement can be very boring if you don't plan ahead and do something constructive with all that free time. Ninety percent of the people interviewed here are still employed in a paying job. Lenny LeShay, at eighty years old still commutes by subway to New York's Garment District for his job. Ivy Browne, at eighty-five, just bought a new car to drive a hundred and five miles to her housekeeping client in Tahoe. Lucille Singleton, at seventy-seven, heads out to her construction job with her tool belt and hard hat almost every morning. The other 10 percent are self-employed, either building their own homes, on the senior sports circuit competing in their chosen sport, or teaching their grandchildren a love of sports early on. We all need to be needed. As Val Orosz put it, "You need something to love in life, whether it's a person, a sport, a hobby, whatever it is, that's what gets you out of bed in the morning."

Diet also plays a key role in successful aging, although not everyone interviewed adheres to a healthy diet. Perhaps good genes does play a role, but for most people it can't hurt to eat a healthful diet. Only about 3 percent of Americans consume at least three daily servings of vegetables and only 28 percent consume at least two daily servings of fruit. Sadly, 59 percent of Americans are overweight. Ralph Hoyle raised an organic garden for seventeen years and attributes his stamina to a daily serving of homegrown, chemical-free vegetables and fruits. Quite a few of the twenty-eight people interviewed are vegetarians. Jack LaLanne has been a vegetarian since the 1940s, when he was labeled as a fanatic, or worse, for his so-called extreme diet. There are self-proclaimed junk food eaters here, but their questionable diets are most likely offset by their exercise routines.

Which brings us to the key factor: exercise. You are never too old to exercise. Being active is critical for seniors. Inactivity is one of the major causes of disability and death from heart disease, diabetes, colon cancer, and high blood pressure. Not only will exercise help you achieve successful aging, it also helps alleviate many conditions such as arthritis. As recently as five years ago, rest was the recommendation for all types of arthritis. Now the advice is just the opposite. Most of the people interviewed here suffer from arthritis. But instead of giving in to the debilitation and living on painkillers, they exercise. Nona Todd was left almost crippled after a car accident. The doctors advised her not to try to walk and put her on a lifetime supply of pain medication. After years of no relief, she flushed the pills down the toilet and is now a serious race walking competitor.

It's also important to have a sense of humor. Positive emotions such as love, caring, purposefulness, and laughter have positive affects on the brain. Norman Cousins calls the value of laughter "internal jogging." Our endorphins go up when we laugh. Laughter and humor prevent us from rigidity of thought and perspective, and have been proven to detoxify medical illness. One reason why my interviews usually ran over the allotted time was due to laughter. All these people have the ability to laugh at themselves and their situations, and they had me laughing along with them. Make sure your last thought of the day is a happy one.

One of our more creative baby boomers, Bob Dylan, wrote these words, which sum up how the people interviewed for this book live their lives:

May your hands always be busy, may your feet always be swift
May your song always be sung, may you stay forever young.

FURTHER READING

Another Country: Navigating the Emotional Terrain of Our Elders, by Mary Pipher. New York: Riverhead Books, 1999.

The Celebration of Life, by Norman Cousins. New York: Harper & Row, 1974

Centenarians: The New Generation, by Belle Boone Beard. Greenwood Press, 1991.

Dare to Be 100, by Walter M. Bortz, M.D. New York: Simon and Schuster, 1996.

Exercise: A Guide from the National Institute of Aging by the Public Information Office. National Institute on Aging, Publication #NIH 99-4258   (800) 222-2225

Growing Old Is Not for Sissies, by Etta Clark. Pomegranate Art Books, 1986.

Just Say Whoa to Aging, by Rosemary Ennis. Santaclara, Utah: Saint George Publishing, (1740 Tamarisk Drive) 801-673-7810

Staying Supple: The Bountiful Pleasures of Streching, John Jerome, Halcottsville, NY: Breakaway Books. 800-548-4348

We Live Too Short and Die Too Long, by Walter M. Bortz, M.D. New York: Bantam Books, 1991.